KV-734-467

A Guide to Dental Radiography

Fourth Edition

RITA A. MASON
Formerly Tutor in Dento-maxillo-facial Radiography
at the Dental School of the London Hospital Medical School

and

SARAH BOURNE
Tutor in Dental Radiography and Superintendent
Radiographer, Dental and Oral Surgery
Imaging Department,
St Bartholomew's and Royal London
School of Medicine and Dentistry,
London

Oxford   New York   Tokyo
OXFORD UNIVERSITY PRESS
1998

Oxford University Press, Great Clarendon Street, Oxford OX2 6DP

Oxford   New York
Athens   Auckland   Bangkok   Bogota   Bombay
Buenos Aires   Calcutta   Cape Town   Dar es Salaam
Delhi   Florence   Hong Kong   Istanbul   Karachi
Kuala Lumpur   Madras   Madrid   Melbourne
Mexico City   Nairobi   Paris   Singapore
Taipei   Tokyo   Toronto   Warsaw

and associated companies in
Berlin   Ibadan

Oxford is a trade mark of Oxford University Press

Published in the United States
by Oxford University Press, Inc., New York

© Rita Mason and Sarah Bourne, 1998

First edition published by John Wright and Sons Ltd 1977
Second edition published by John Wright and Sons Ltd 1982
Third edition published by Butterworths 1998

All rights reserved. No part of this publication may be
reproduced, stored in a retrieval system, or transmitted, in any
form or by any means, without the prior permission in writing of Oxford
University Press. Within the UK, exceptions are allowed in respect of any
fair dealing for the purpose of research or private study, or criticism or
review, as permitted under the Copyright, Designs and Patents Act, 1988, or
in the case of reprographic reproduction in accordance with the terms of
licences issued by the Copyright Licensing Agency. Enquiries concerning
reproduction outside those terms and in other countries should be sent to
the Rights Department, Oxford University Press, at the address above.

This book is sold subject to the condition that it shall not,
by way of trade or otherwise, be lent, re-sold, hired out, or otherwise
circulated without the publisher's prior consent in any form of binding
or cover other than that in which it is published and without a similar
condition including this condition being imposed
on the subsequent purchaser.

A catalogue record for this book is available from the British Library

Library of Congress Cataloging in Publication Data
Mason, Rita A.
A guide to dental radiography / Rita Mason and Sarah Bourne.—
4th ed.
(Oxford medical publications)
Includes bibliographical references and index.
1. Teeth—Radiography.   I. Bourne, Sarah.   II. Title.
III. Series.
[DNLM: 1. Radiography, Dental—methods.   WN 230 M411g 1998]
RK309.M38   1988   617.6'07572—dc21   97–28365

ISBN 0 19 262672 8 (Hbk)
0 19 262671 X (Pbk)

Typeset by
EXPO Holdings, Malaysia

Printed in Great Britain by
The Bath Press, Avon

SBRLSMD

CLASS MARK	WN230 MAS 1998
CIRC TYPE	BMBC 06/99
SUPPLIER	£32.50
BINDING	

Foreword

Dr Malcolm I. Coombs
Head – Oral Diagnosis and Radiology
    Oral and Maxillofacial Surgery
The University of Sydney, Australia

It is indeed a privilege and pleasure to write the foreword to this, the fourth edition of *A Guide to Dental Radiography*. Rita and I were weaned on radiology as our fathers 'Harry' Coombs and Sydney Blackman were both pioneers in establishing the teaching of Radiology in learning institutions in the United Kingdom. However, our own paths were only destined to cross during the Röntgen Centenary Congress in Birmingham in 1995. It was here we had the opportunity to spend several hours together and discuss our inheritance and how our respective careers had developed from those early beginnings. It is most gratifying to see that Rita has a successor in Sarah Bourne who is dedicated to continuing the development of this subject and has collaborated in the writing of this edition.

As a teacher of Dental Radiology it is essential to have a reference text which is simple and straightforward for students to comprehend. This book fulfills the criteria required as it offers ease of reading and understanding with step-by-step guidelines. Over the past twenty years this text has been the mainstay for the teaching of Dental Radiography to both under- and postgraduate students from a range of disciplines in many institutions around the world.

Dentomaxillofacial radiology is considered 'the hub' of the diagnostic wheel which embraces all disciplines of dentistry. It is essential that the clinician be fully aware of all aspects of radiology to utilize this very important diagnostic aid for the benefit of the patient. It is very refreshing to see that this latest edition has retained the easy to handle and read format with key areas emphasized. In a day and age when computers are becoming the norm the basic principles of radiography remain the same. The interpretation of a radiographic image, whether it be from a film or computer screen is still dependent upon these basic principles which the authors have continued to reinforce.

This edition has built upon the past with the future in mind and will continue to be one of the quality texts used in the teaching of dental radiology to the dental and allied professions. I am delighted to have had the opportunity to peruse this book prior to printing and look forward to its availability for use in our curriculum here in Sydney, Australia.

Preface

It is rewarding to know that 20 years after the publication of the first edition in 1977, there is still a need for a practical book on dental radiography.

The previous editions have been in the Dental Practitioners' Handbook series and this new edition follows that tradition.

It is now statutory for the dental graduate to undertake a Vocational Training Scheme for General Dental Practice, when they have to confront the X-ray apparatus on their own and do their own problem-solving.

Graham Hooper, in Bristol, who takes his radiographs in the working position, encouraged us to help the dentist in practice, by including the adaptation necessary to undertake the recognized intra-oral techniques in this situation. He has also given practical help, including allowing us a 'photocall' in his surgery and providing intra-oral radiographic examples.

The advent of computerization with the digital image is another challenge. It enables the image to be enhanced but still cannot manipulate the projection.

It was fortunate that Sarah Bourne who was Rita Mason's successor in the academic appointment of Tutor in Dental Radiography, (at the now St Bartholomew's and Royal London School of Medicine and Dentistry), agreed to be co-author for this new edition. In particular, Sarah has covered advances in dental panoramic tomography and the support for implantology as well as other specialized techniques.

The anatomical variations of the dental arches are addressed by Dr Anita Sengupta, lecturer in Dental Anatomy at the Medical School at Bristol University, and she also focuses on how this relates to the difficulty of applying 'standard' techniques.

Quality assurance is of increasing importance to improve the overall standards of dental radiography, and in so doing, minimize the ionizing radiation dosage by reducing retakes.

The protection chapter as before, is of course a high priority including the latest recommendations for General Dental Practice.

Particular thanks must go to Keith Horner for his generosity in giving the theoretical background information for the digitizing chapter, and Andrew Hall at the Bristol Dental Hospital and School for his practical input.

Also from the Dental Hospital and School in Bristol thanks must go to Professor Richard Elderton, for allowing access to his department and staff for help using the Digora digital apparatus. Thanks to all for their cooperation.

Most of all, John Bunn the Superintendent Radiographer gave Rita help in many ways, from giving access to the X-ray department to proofreading (with constructive advice), and even helping choose and position figures into the text.

Dr Heather Andrews and Dr Jane Luker from the Radiology Departments of the United Bristol Hospitals Trust have been invaluable, in particular for giving examples of specialized techniques associated with the salivary glands, in particular sialography. Dr Martin Morse and Janet Wheeler of the Nuclear Medical Imaging Department at Frenchay Hospital also deserve our thanks for their imaging contributions and advice for the same chapter.

Liz Pitcher of the medical physics department at the Bristol General Hospital updated the Protection chapter working from the first draft written by the late Derek Gifford from the same department and as in previous editions John Hewitt of the NRPB has been an excellent referee. He also pointed us in the right direction for obtaining permission to reproduce many items from their publications. The Regional Dental Officer, John Lucia, gave the benefit of his experience pointing out the particular areas of omissions.

Last but certainly not least, from the Bristol fraternity, Liz Hurst, the medical illustrator whose photographs and diagrams have been essential in helping to demonstrate so much of the purpose of the book.

John Richards, as in the previous editions, gave advice and practical help for the text and illustrations in the endodontic section. Gary Pollock, lecturer in Prosthetic Dentistry, also at St. Bartholomew's and Royal London School of Medicine and Dentistry has given Sarah every possible support and help with the Implant chapter in particular.

The audio-visual department from the School has again been invaluable.

On the hospital side, Sarah has had the support of the Medical Imaging Departments with images for illustration of CTs, and Ultrasound. Jane Schwiezo supplied the MRI images, and Mark Sewell gave information and images in radio-isotopes.

Professor NJD Smith kindly gave an example of the Orthophos as applied in Sialography.

Peter Hirschmann, editor of the Journal of the International Association of Dento-maxillofacial Radiology, gave permission to use digital examples from the Journal, with access to Stockton Press and the authors. He has also given us the benefit of his advice.

Dr Malcolm Coombs, uniquely qualified in radiography as well as dentistry, gave his opinion and suggestions in some of the more difficult and contentious areas and kindly offered to write the Foreword.

Many firms have been very co-operative enabling us to copy illustrations from brochures or giving extra product slides. In particular Siemens gave us digital images through Paul Want at Sident. Harold Trunley of Clark Dental, similarly gave images from Schick CCD with the permission to use the illustrations from the brochure. Peter Taylor of Royston Scientific has also given invaluable support with the Digora as has Dave Robinson from Dentaleez.

Geoff Sparrow and John Collins of Belmont Equipment Corporation gave permission to use their new Belray brochure, and Dennis Burstow of Densply contributed with extra illustrations of Oralix timers and Rinn products, plus the permission to use and adapt diagrams.

Alan Kiem of Keystone gave us the excellent diagram of the Discovery tube head.

John MacMahon from Kodak has made available all the practical publications at his disposal, and we thank him for his support and cooperation.

Sarah wishes to thank her colleagues in the Dental Institute for being so patient over the last year, as well as her radiographic colleagues for their help and suggestions as without their support and understanding she could never have undertaken this project.

Professor Robert Langlais deserves special mention for his ongoing support and advice. His help has been invaluable.

Finally, thanks to the staff of the Oxford University Press for their help and encouragement with this new edition.

Bristol and London   R.M
October 1997   S.B

Contents

This book is dedicated to the memory of Professor Sydney Blackman, who would be proud to know that the high standards he set in dental radiography over fifty years ago are still maintained today and continue to evolve within the new technology.

Introduction

This new edition of the *Guide to Dental Radiography*, as the previous editions, has been written by radiographers whose specialty is dental radiography. It is a book which covers the practical aspects of dental imaging as well as incorporating specialized techniques, and can be seen as complementary to general radiography and dental radiology books.

Dental graduates need to fulfill a vocational training scheme before embarking on their careers, and so are faced with having to take their own radiographs and quality assurance. There are several chapters discussing the two intra-oral techniques with the advantages and disadvantages to both. The chapter on radiation protection has been updated and includes the current guidelines on standards of dental radiography as well as the Ionizing Radiations Regulations core of knowledge. Quality Assurance is of increasing importance to improve standards so these chapters will also help those who have been in practice for a while and wish to maintain and update their skills as part of continuing their professional development. There have been advances in planning and support for implants and a chapter has been included to cover this, giving advantages and disadvantages of all the current techniques to aid practitioners.

This book is ideal for dental auxillaries who are being trained or who have been trained to undertake dental radiography for their dentist, and for dental therapists who are able to treat their own patients under the prescriptive regulations of dental practice. There is an ever increasing demand for dental radiographs in District General Hospitals and with the chapter on anatomical variations of the dental arches, radiographers who are not completely at ease with the mysteries of dental techniques (or anyone who is required to produce these images) will find the book useful.

The chapter on Dental Panoramic Tomography will be essential to anyone who has never encountered this technique before. The applications, advantages, and disadvantages are discussed as well as the technique and the pitfalls.

Most radiographers will be experienced in facial bone radiography and indications for each view have been included to help choose the most relevant radiograph for the patients' problem. The chapter on specialized techniques will be of interest to practitioners as well as the maxillo-facial surgeon.

This book is also designed for the undergraduate, in dentistry and radiography, and can be regarded as a teaching aid and a reference with suggestions to further reading at the end of each chapter.

1 Radiation protection

1.1 INTRODUCTION

The radiograph is one of the most valuable diagnostic tools available in the practice of dentistry. It is an image of the teeth and surrounding tissues produced by X-rays and may be a chemically produced or digital image. However, ionizing radiation, such as X-rays, interacts with living tissue by the absorption of radiation energy into the tissues. This may cause damage either through chemical or molecular changes, both of which can be produced almost immediately. On the other hand, biological changes or damage can become manifest over a very long period of time — sometimes decades.

New facts on the effects of ionizing radiation — which can become apparent 5–30 years following the initial dosage — are continuously being recognized. Nevertheless, radiographs are of considerable value as diagnostic tools and, when the appropriate measures are observed, they act as an essential adjunct to dentistry, requiring only a small radiation dose.

There are regulations and recommendations which provide an appropriate standard of protection without unduly limiting the beneficial practice.

1.1.1 International Commission on Radiation Protection (ICRP) 26

These regulations (ICRP 1977) have three basic principles:

- justification
- optimization
- limitation.

The regulations set out to control the damage caused by all ionization radiations, including X-rays, measuring their harm to living tissue in recognized international units.

Key points

1. Radiographs, valuable diagnostic tool
2. Ionizing radiation can cause damage to human tissue
3. Regulations, essential
   — justification
   — optimization
   — limitation

It should also be realized that we live in an environment where we are exposed to natural background radiation of both cosmic and terrestrial origin. Within the UK there will be regional differences. For example, the level of terrestrial radiation (radon) in Cornwall is six times higher than in London (Fig. 1.1).

(a)

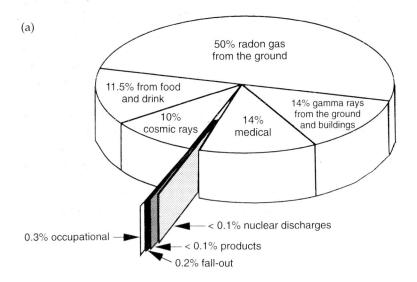

50% radon gas
from the ground

11.5% from food
and drink

10%
cosmic rays

14%
medical

14% gamma rays
from the ground
and buildings

< 0.1% nuclear discharges

0.3% occupational

< 0.1% products

0.2% fall-out

(b)

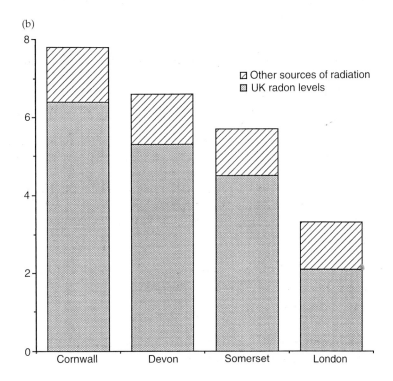

Other sources of radiation
UK radon levels

Cornwall　　Devon　　Somerset　　London

Fig. 1.1　(a) Average annual radiation dose equivalent, received by the population in the UK (2.6 mSv); (b) Differences of radon levels in some areas of the UK (NRPB 1994*a*).

1.2 THE PHYSICAL NATURE OF X-RAYS

The regulations governing the use of X-rays are necessary because of their potential for causing harm. X-rays are a form of electromagnetic radiation, as are light and radiowaves. They are characterized by short wavelengths and high energy. Consequently, as the rays pass through matter they transfer energy. This energy causes electrons to be released from their orbital shells, resulting in the production of an ion — hence the term 'ionizing radiation'. During radiation exposure it is the production of these ionization events that causes the majority of immediate chemical changes in tissue.

The critical molecules for the radiation damage processes are believed to be proteins (such as enzymes) and nuclear acids (principally DNA).

The high energy of X-rays enables them to pass through most solid objects to a variable degree. The intensity of the radiation beam continues to fall as it passes through tissue, but at any given depth a residual beam always remains. It is this differential attenuation of X-radiation in matter that is utilized in the production of diagnostic radiographs (Fig. 1.2).

1.3 FACTORS CONCERNED WITH IONIZING RADIATION DOSAGE

All units of ionizing radiation dosage are measured using the Systeme Internationale (SI) units.

The effect of ionizing radiation on tissue depends on radiation energy. X-rays are not the only form of ionizing radiation. Other types include protons and alpha particles.

The absorbed dose on the surface of the patient is not just related to the incidence of the absorbed dose in air, but must also take into account the difference in the absorbing medium. This is called the weighting factor (W) and depends on the relative biological effectiveness (RBE) of the radiation in inducing stochastic effects at low doses: in other words, how quickly the energy is absorbed and, thus, causes biological damage.

1. *Absorbed dose* (D) is the amount of radiation energy absorbed per unit mass of tissue. This is measured in Grays.

1 Gray (Gy) = 1 J/kg (joules/kilogram)

2. *Equivalent dose* (H) takes into account the effect of the type of radiation and is measured in Sieverts (Sv).

Key points

1. X-rays, part of electromagnetic radiation
2. X-rays transfer energy when they pass through matter
3. X-rays cause chemical damage in tissue
4. Damage molecules
   — proteins
   — nuclear acids (DNA)
5. Differential attentuation of X-ray beam utilized for radiographs

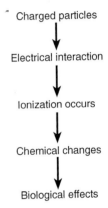

Charged particles

↓

Electrical interaction

↓

Ionization occurs

↓

Chemical changes

↓

Biological effects

Fig. 1.2 Ionizing radiation and tissue. (NRPB 1990)

X-rays are radiation type R.
The weighting factor for R = 1
$$\therefore W_R = 1$$
$$\therefore \text{Equivalent dose (H)} = W_R D = 1 \times D$$
$$\therefore H \text{ (equivalent dose: Sieverts)} = D \text{ (absorbed dose in tissue: Grays)}$$

- For general dental practice and hospital application 1 Sv = 1 Gy.
- The Sievert is such a large unit that, for medical applications, dose is measured in milliSieverts (mSv) and microSieverts (μSv)
- In dental and maxillo-facial radiography the dose is calculated by simulating the procedures using tissue equivalent phantom heads to which dosemeters have been applied.

3. *Effective dose.* In order to compare the relative doses from different X-ray examinations the concept of effective dose equivalents has been introduced. For a particular examination the effective dose equivalent (H_E) is the dose which, if given to the whole body, would give the same risks of mortality as the non-uniform dose resulting from the examination in question.

There are weighting factors for each organ:

	Weighting factor (W_R)
Gonads	0.20
Bone marrow	0.12
Colon	0.12
Lung	0.12
Stomach	0.12
Bladder	0.05
Breast	0.05
Liver	0.05
Oesophagus	0.05
Thyroid	0.05
Skin	0.01
Bone surfaces	0.01
Remainder	0.05

Prior to ICRP 60 an alternative unit called the effective dose equivalent was used which used slightly different weighting factors (Fig. 1.3).

4. *Collective effective dose.* This is the collective dose for all people × the dose per particular examination. The radiation dose per individual in having a dental radiographic examination is small, but the proportion of the population who undergo this procedure regularly and in their dentist's surgery is relatively large, so it cannot be disregarded. (Fig. 1.4)

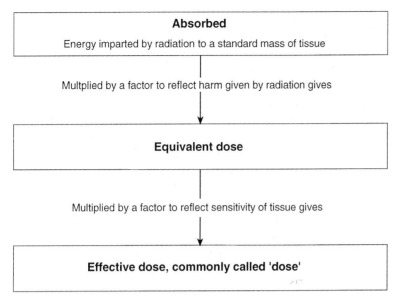

Fig. 1.3   Hierarchy of doses, taking harm and sensitivity into account. (NRPB 1994*b*)

UK annual collective dose

Source of exposure	UK annual collective dose (man Sv)
All dental radiography (patients)	200
All medical diagnostic radiology (patients)	20,000
Nuclear medicine (patients)	1,400
All natural sources	127,000
All occupational exposure	430

*Radiology Standards for Primary Care
from a range of sources for 1991*

Fig. 1.4   Annual collective doses from a range of sources for the year 1991 ref NRPB Guidelines on Radiological Standards for Primary Dental Care 1994.

On the other hand, it is very small compared to radiation from natural sources (NRPB 1994*c*). (Weighting factor for background radiation (radon) = 20)

1.4   BIOLOGICAL AND DETRIMENTAL EFFECTS OF RADIATION

There are various harmful effects of ionizing radiation which have been observed over a hundred years of use. They are subdivided as follows:

(a) somatic — which occur in the individual exposed;
(b) genetic — which occur in descendants of the individual exposed.

1.4.1   Somatic effects

1. *Deterministic*: the severity of the radiation effect will increase with the dose received, but there is a threshold dose below which this effect does not occur, or there is no probability or chance of the effect occurring.

Deterministic effects are entirely somatic. The risks of these effects have been quantified by monitoring populations exposed to radiation, for example, atomic bomb survivors. Of course, in the early days of radiography, before the hazards of ionizing radiation were properly understood, there were many mishaps and errors in technique, so the effects of X-rays were seen quite quickly. Nowadays such effects are not seen due to the improved safety standards.

- Lower doses repeated over a long period of time can produce damage to skin, including epilation.
- The eyes are very sensitive and repeated small doses can cause point opacities, leading to cataracts.
- Natural biological repair, as is the case with cataracts and skin ulceration, means that there is not a direct linear relationship between dose and effect.

In fact, eyes are *the* most sensitive part of the body. Therefore it is important that the dose to the eyes is as low as possible.

2. *Non-deterministic or stochastic*: where there is no threshold dose below which no radiation effect occurs. The risk or probability of the effect occurring is assessed to increase linearly with the dose received. The magnitude and nature of the induced damage increases with several factors:

(a) the radiation dose;
(b) the rate at which the dose is given;
(c) the volume of tissue irradiated;
(d) the way the radiation deposits its energy.

Key points (Fig. 1.5)

Detrimental effects of X-rays
1. Somatic—occurs in individuals
2. Genetic—occurs in descendants
3. Deterministic—entirely somatic
   — there is a threshold dose below which effects do not occur
   — there is biological repair
4. Non-deterministic—no threshold dose
   — risk increases with linear dosage
   — cancer induction and genetic changes in chromosomes: can produce mutations
5. If regulations abided by—small, compared to naturally occurring abnormalities

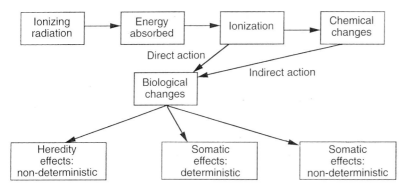

Fig. 1.5 The sequence of events when radiation is absorbed by a biological medium.

The damage caused by the radiation at low doses is expressed as 'cancer induction', or the 'hereditary' or 'genetic' effect, and is thought to be the result of a cell being damaged and changing function, which may lead to carcinogenesis after a latent period of several years. Carcinogenesis is often the result when large sections of the body are irradiated.

New facts on the stochastic effects of ionizing radiation are continuously being recognized. As has already been stated effects can be seen 5–30 years following the initial dosage.

Information on carcinogenic (as well as genetic effects) has been gained from observation of the survivors of the Hiroshima and Nagasaki nuclear bombs, and from biological experiments.

1.4.2 Genetic effects

There are other changes produced by radiation which do not affect the health of the irradiated person and yet, which, in the long run, have deleterious effects. These changes may be produced in chromosomes when male or female gonads are irradiated. These hereditary effects could produce mutations which affect the fetus, causing physical or mental handicap.

1. The risks are small compared to naturally occurring abnormalities. Nevertheless it is desirable to keep irradiation of the gonads to a minimum. In the dental field the risk is extremely small, as the 1994 Guidelines on Radiology Standards for Primary Dental Care state. Dosages are small and the X-ray beam is seldom directed towards the gonads.

2. Special care is needed in radiography during pregnancy — as much for the reassurance of the patients as for any other reason. During the most sensitive period of pregnancy, from the 8th to

15th week, it is generally considered that there should be a reduction of radiation, if at all possible, despite the fact that any dose to the fetus in dental radiography is likely to be of the order of microsieverts.

3. As with all radiographic examinations, investigations must be justified. In 1993 the National Radiological Protection Board (NRPB) published a statement that while the current advice draws upon data published since 1985, the main objective is unchanged — keeping unnecessary exposure to a minimum. However, in the case of inadvertent exposure, with likely dose thresholds, there is no substantial risk for the individual pregnancy regarding the well-being of the fetus, and termination would not be advised.

1.5   RISK FACTORS

Background radiation is the greatest source of radiation dose received by the majority of the population during their lifetime. (See Fig. 1.1). In the UK, the average dose received is about 2.6 mSv per annum. It is useful to look at the current risk factors to the general population in normal daily life and the overall illness risks.

At this time all the data is being re-examined and will lead to a lower level of risk limitation and lower dose limits. Below are the factors as they are currently understood.

Taking the recommended upper limit of constraints as 1 mSv, the equivalent risks are:

Driving a car for 6 months
Smoking 10 cigarettes a day for 4 days
Travelling 12 500 miles by air
Skiing for 1 hour

The current risk factors for getting the following disease:

For the working population

Fatal cancer	4.0×10^2	1 in 25 000 mSv[1]
Non-fatal cancer	0.9×10^2 Sv	1 in 111 000 mSv[1]
Genetic effects	0.6×10^2 Sv	1 in 167 000 mSv[1]
Total	5.5×10^2 Sv[1]	1 in 18 000 mSv[1]

For general population

Total	7.2×10^2 Sv[1]	1 in 14 000 mSv[1]

It is useful to compare effective doses between different radiographic examinations:

Type of examination		*Effective dose equivalents (H_E) per X-ray examination (in manSieverts)*
Lumber spine		2.15
Chest		0.05
Skull		0.15
Abdomen		1.39
Barium enema		7.69
Computed tomographic examination		
Head		3.5
Cervical spine		1.9
Doses from dental radiography		
Intra-oral	2	0.02
Extra-oral	2	0.03
Dental panaromic tomography	1	0.08

1.6   LEGISLATION

The Health and Safety Executive has suggested that the maximum acceptable risks to the population are as follows:

(a) 1 in 10 000 for the public;
(b) 1 in 1000 for workers.

The dose limits for staff and members of the public are based on these maximum risks.

The current protection legislation is based on the recommendations of the International Commission on Radiation Protection as published in ICRP 60 (ICRP 1991) and ICRP 26 (ICRP 1977). These recommendations have three general principles:

1. No practice shall be adopted unless its introduction produces a positive net benefit.

2. All exposures shall be kept as low as reasonably achievable (ALARA principle) — economic and social factors being taken into account. In UK law this is taken to mean as low as reasonably practicable (ALARP).

3. The dose equivalent to individuals shall not exceed the limits recommended for the appropriate circumstances by the Commission.

These recommendations are implemented in the UK through two main regulations:

1. Protection of staff and members of the public

• The Ionizing Radiations Regulations (IRR) 1985 (SI no. 133) came into effect from 1986. This is part of the Health and Safety at Work Act, 1974. It is obligatory for every practitioner to comply with these regulations.

2. Protection for the patient

• Protection of Persons Undergoing Medical Examination or Treatment (**POPUMET**) came into effect through the Ionizing Radiation Regulations (IRR) 1988 (SI no. 778).

The clinical and physical directing of ionizing radiation should be in accordance with regulations and guidelines discussed below.

• The patient is also protected by a legal obligation, as imposed by IRR 1988. With regard to the training of practitioners and their acquisition of a 'Core of Knowledge':

    (a) The dentist may have qualified before ionizing radiation risks were fully appreciated. Protection and ionizing radiation risks are now included in the dental curriculum, so dentists qualifying before 1988 have to prove that they have attended a supplementary course.

    (b) The 1994 Guidelines on Radiology Standards for Primary Dental Care recommend that by 1998 dental radiology should be a more integral and necessary part of the undergraduate curriculum, with a specific examination and test of practical competence.

IRR 1985 and IRR 1988 are enforced by the Health and Safety Executive, except for Regulation 4 of IRR 1985.

The Department of Health has responsibility for the application of this particular regulation.

Regulation 4 includes guidelines for dentists in the form of a Code of Practice. This Code of Practice aims to ensure the safe use of radiation in a dental practice, both for the workers and the patients. Practitioners must work within the dose limits and abide by the regulations.

1.6.1   Dose limits

Dose Limits for workers and the general public

The dose limits quoted in IRR 1985 are considerably below any threshold dose. The primary aim of the regulations is to maintain conditions whereby any doses received by workers or the general public are below levels which might give rise to any ionization radiation effects.

Dose limit for the public
It is recommended that the dose should be 2.5 mSv

Dose limits for workers

Whole body	50 mSv
Eyes	150 mSv
Extremities and organs	500 mSv
Fetal gestation	10 mSv

• These limits are likely to be reduced, as we are working towards proposed new regulations which would recommend that:

(1) the dose limit for the general public would be lowered to 1 mSv per year;

(2) the dosage for workers would be reduced so that over 5 years it would not exceed 100 mSv.

It follows that if the limit of 50 mSv is reached in a year, the limit for succeeding years will be greatly reduced.

Pregnant staff: once pregnancy is declared, the exposure of the pregnant woman should be further restricted so as to limit the additional effective dose to the fetus to 10 mSv, but reducing it towards the proposed new dose limit of 1 mSv.

Dose limits for the patient

The patient cannot avoid exposure to the primary beam. There is no dose limit but the ALARA or ALARP principle of course applies. The dental practitioner has the responsibility to be properly trained to direct medical exposure and to be aware of all radiographic examinations undertaken.

1.6.2   IRR 1985

IRR 1985 affects the dental practitioner in the following areas.

1. The use of ionizing radiation must be notified to the Health and Safety Executive.

2. Every user must appoint a radiation protection supervisor. Who is a designated dentist working within the practice who has acquired the core of knowledge.

3. Every user must produce local rules to ensure the safe use of ionizing radiation in the dental practice. These are to be read by all members of staff.

4. Quality control methods should be employed on a regular basis.

The role of a radiation protection adviser and supervisor

The Health and Safety Executive have allowed general dental practice to be exempted from the need to appoint a radiation protection adviser, a medical physicist, so long as:

(1) the terms of Regulation 10 are being observed — that is, a controlled area has been defined and designated and this is not entered by anyone except the patient;

(2) the work-load in any week does not exceed 30 mA minutes in dental radiography (about 300 films) or 150 mA minutes in dental panoramic radiography (about 50 films) (in large group practices, this limit applies to each dental X-ray set);

(3) where cephalometry is not undertaken.

When appointed, the radiation protection adviser or supervisor must be consulted on and responsible for the following matters:

- restriction of exposure
- maintenance of apparatus
- identification of controlled areas
- drawing up of local rules
- dosimetry and monitoring
- selection of the successive Radiation Protection Supervisor
- training
- suspected high exposures

The radiation protection supervisor has managerial responsibility to:

(1) draft and display local rules;

(2) ensure compliance with local rules;

(3) ensure compliance with the IRR 1985 and 1988 and the Approved Code of Practice (ACOP).

1. *Restriction of exposure*: designed to reduce the patient dose by:

(a) only carrying out appropriate examinations;
(b) optimizing doses if an examination is done.

2. *Maintenance of apparatus*: obligatory servicing every 3 years (Regulation 33 (1), IRR 1985).

3. *Identification of controlled areas*: and restricted access to controlled areas.

4. Where the instantaneous dose exceeds 7.5 μSvh^{-1} the controlled area extends to a distance of 1.0 m for sets operating up to 70 kV and

1.5 m for sets operating above 70 kV (Fig. 1.6). The advice of a radiation protection adviser is to be recommended initially, to help with the regulations regarding the setting up of a controlled area.

4. *Drawing up of local rules*: these should include:
   (a) a description and plan of the controlled area, and the procedure for determining its extent and when it is operational;
   (b) the procedure for restricting access to the controlled area;
   (c) the names and telephone numbers of the radiation protection adviser (if required) and of the radiation protection supervisor;
   (d) the details of any system of work which may be necessary in special circumstances, such as when the X-ray unit is being operated by a X-ray service engineer;
   (e) a possible procedure if a patient is unable to co-operate, for example, a very young child or a patient with a physical handicap;
   (f) quality control methods to be used on a regular basis;
   (g) the date.

It could be a criminal offence to fail to observe the local rules; if it is necessary to alter the working practice, any change must be reflected in the local rules.

5. *Dosimetry and monitoring*:
   (a) Personal monitoring — while it is to be recommended that monitoring devices should be worn by all staff and checked regularly, this is generally necessary only when the work-load exceeds 150 films per week.

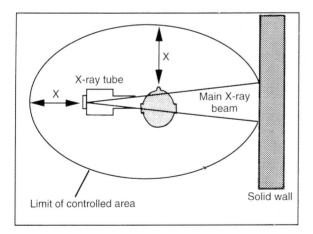

Fig. 1.6 Diagram of a controlled area which may be defined as extending to distance 'x'. (NRPB 1995). x = 1.0 m for sets operating up to 70 kV, or 1.5 m for sets operating above 70 kV and within the main X-ray beam until it has been sufficiency attenuated by distance or absorption.

(b)   Quality Control — to produce diagnostic radiographs with the minimum radiation to the patient and in the most cost-effective way.

6. *Selection of radiation protection supervisors*: must have appropriate training to include the 'Core of Knowledge'.

7. *Training*: the radiation protection supervisor is also responsible for ensuring that all staff, dentists, or dental auxiliaries have received approved instruction both in the X-ray techniques employed and/or in suitable radiation protection procedures. Staff is divided into two categories:
  (a)   those clinically directing (for whom IRR 1988 has particular relevance);
  (b)   those physically directing.

The dentist usually fulfils both roles but, increasingly, with the training of dental auxiliaries, he/she may only perform the first.

8. *Suspected high exposures*: in the unfortunate event of one occurring, the Health and Safety Executive must be called to investigate.

  In the case of a radiation accident to an employee or patient, the radiation protection adviser must be informed immediately. A written statement must be taken from the operator and signed as soon as possible. Any personal monitors should be sent off immediately for measurement and, if sufficiently high, the Department of Health and the Health and Safety Executive must be informed. The person or persons involved should be informed of the dose they have received and counselled. Appropriate medical advice should be sought, if necessary.

1.7   PRACTICAL ASPECTS OF X-RAY PROTECTION IRR 1985 AND 1988, AND THE APPROVED CODE OF PRACTICE

The need to avoid unnecessary exposure to radiation applies both to the patient and to the operator. However, while the operator must avoid totally any exposure to the primary beam, the patient cannot avoid exposure to it. For both, exposure to secondary or scattered radiation must be minimized.

1.7.1   Protection for the operators and staff working in the practice

The first important condition for maintaining satisfactory standards of radiation protection in the dental practice is to ensure that the necessary administrative structure is in place. This will define who has responsibility for what, and how.

Radiation protection can be regarded as having four main elements:

1. Dose limits. This has been covered earlier in the chapter.

2. Personal monitoring
This is only necessary in high work-load practice.
- It must be emphasized that if monitoring badges are worn, and if any of the dose limits are approached by a member of the staff, then the arrangements for radiation protection in the practice should be reviewed instantly, as a matter of urgency.

Staff tend to assume that protective measures, as listed in the local rules provided by the employer, will, in themselves, provide sufficient protection. In fact, it is the way in which the procedures are implemented by the staff that determines the levels of dose that they and their patients will receive.

3. Physical barriers
These include some of the simplest and most effective protection measures.

(a) *Distance*
Radiation intensity decreases with the square of the distance from the source. Doubling the distance from the tube reduces the dose which may be received to a quarter. Always stand at least 1.5 m from the X-ray beam in any direction, preferably behind the X-ray tube head, for X-ray apparatus operating at 70 kV.

Never hold the film in the patient's mouth.

(b) *Barriers — fixed and mobile*
Examples include:
- walls and doors
- floors and ceilings
- protective screens
- lead gloves, aprons, gonad shields, and such like.

Ideally, there should be a remote controlled exposure panel, behind a protective barrier that incorporates 0.5 mm of lead. Failing that, if the control panel is behind the X-ray apparatus column there should be a 2 m cable on the timer — enough for the operator to be outside the controlled area. If there is insufficient space to achieve the required distance, then a protective barrier must be used.

4. Familiarity with X-ray techniques
Adequate training should be given to staff to ensure competence in, and confidence with, radiographic procedures.

If at all possible, eye contact should be maintained with the patient during X-ray examination. Apart from giving the patient reassurance,

Key points

Protection of the operator
1. Personal monitoring
2. Stand 1.5 m away from, and at right angles to, the primary beam
3. If work-load demands, or lack of room, stand behind a lead shield of 0.5 mm
4. Do not hold the film in the patient's mouth
5. Do not hold the patient during exposure
6. Competence in radiographic techniques— to avoid unnecessary retakes

it allows the operator to monitor the patient for movement and so avoid unnecessary radiation due to a retake.

The time and motion procedures detailed in Chapter 6 should also be employed.

1.7.2 Protection for the patient

The patient receives two types of radiation. Primary radiation — from the primary or 'useful' beam emerging from the X-ray tube; and secondary radiation. These doses depend not only on the exposure given to the patient in the area of treatment, but also upon the irradiated volume of tissue within the primary beam.

General protective amount of secondary radiation received measures include:

1. No radiograph should be taken without specific justification from the dentist.

2. Every dentist is responsible for each exposure and must be prepared to justify its clinical necessity — that is, he or she *clinically directs.*

3. Even when the radiographs are undertaken by a trained dental auxiliary, the dentist is still responsible in the same way.

Practical ways of minimizing the exposure dose from the primary beam

1. Reduce the exposure as much as possible in intra-oral radiography, by using the fastest film consistent with good diagnostic quality — speed D or E. In extra-oral radiography, use intensifying screens — the fastest that can provide the necessary resolution (rare-earth screens if possible). (Fig. 1.7)

2. With apparatus that incorporates variable kV and mA, ensure that the correct exposure factors are chosen. Sometimes the timer is the only variable control — be sure this is correctly set.

3. The operator — dentist, radiographer, or dental auxiliary — must have received approved training and be practically competent — to ensure that the radiographic technique is well chosen and properly executed in order to be diagnostic, and to avoid retakes.

4. Reliable and consistent processing is essential for the production of high-quality radiographs, and quality control must be vigorously applied. Radiographs that might have been of good diagnostic value can be ruined in processing. (Processing is one area

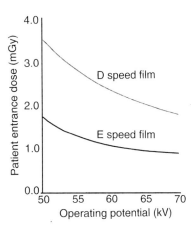

Fig. 1.7 Graph showing differing radiation doses for D and E speed films. (NRPB 1995)

in general dental practice often found to be below an acceptable level.)

5. If there is a choice of collimator, ensure that the correct device is attached to the X-ray tube.

6. Film holders and/or custom-made bitewing films should be used at all times to save the patient holding the film and receiving both primary and secondary radiation.

How to minimize exposure to secondary radiation

Tissue irradiated by the primary beam emits secondary or 'scattered' radiation from the patient in all directions. This characteristic of secondary radiation makes it, in some ways, more difficult to protect against than primary radiation, although its intensity and energy is much lower.

The critical parts of the body that require protection against scatter radiation are the gonads and, in pregnancy, the fetus.

Recent surveys have shown that during dental radiography only a negligible radiation dose is received by the gonads, but special care should be taken when the beam is directed to this area. Fortunately, scattered radiation is much less penetrating than the primary beam, and an apron with lead content equivalent to 0.25 mm offers more than adequate protection.

Lead aprons   The 1994 Guidelines on Radiation Standards for Primary Dental Care (NRPB 1994c) cover this area thoroughly and conclude that there is no justification for the routine use of lead aprons for dental radiography.

Whilst this may be true in an ideal world, when the standards aspired to in the guidelines have been achieved, it would still perhaps be advisable to keep a lead apron on the premises. Wearing a lead apron for X-ray dental examinations reassures the patient that the dentist is taking proper care and attention. This is important in view of public concern and media coverage about the hazards of ionizing radiation.

The authors consider that lead aprons should be offered to all patients, perhaps with an explanation of the current thinking that it is no longer of paramount importance. In particular, a lead apron should be used for certain views, for example, upper incisors and for the following:

(a) pregnant women;

(b) women of child bearing age;

(c) any person supporting a child or adult patient and who will, inevitably therefore, be in the controlled area. These exceptional circumstances must be included in the local rules. The supporting person should *never* be a member of staff.

Key points

Protection for the patient
1. Do not irradiate unless clinically necessary
2. Use film holders for both paralleling and bisecting angle techniques
3. Choose the appropriate technique for the area under examination
4. Assess the anatomical and management limitations of the patient
5. Set exposure times correctly
6. Use the fastest film consistent with good quality
7. Use intensifying screens for extra-oral examinations
8. Processing facilities should be constantly monitored— quality control
9. Lead apron for the patient if appropriate

Key points

Protection for members of the public
1. Never allowed in controlled area
2. Design of room *vis-à-vis* position of apparatus
3. X-ray beam directed to outside wall
4. Hazard lights and signs on door

Protection for members of the public

Preventing entry into a controlled area

- The appropriate warning signs, as specified in British Standard (BS) 510, must be displayed outside the door of the dental surgery or X-ray room to indicate if one is entering a controlled area.
- No one, other than the patient may remain within a controlled area when an exposure is being made.

Most modern dental X-ray units emit an audible warning when the tube is energized.

- An essential condition for the use of X-ray equipment in dental practice is that only one X-ray tube can be energized at one time in the same room.

Direction and penetration of radiation beam

The positioning of the dental X-ray equipment is important in the interests of the general public. If enough care is not taken in the design of the room in which the dental X-ray set is situated, radiation may penetrate into adjacent rooms, including those above and below the installation.

Consider the hazard to people working in these rooms who are in the direct path of the primary beam. If the work-load is sufficiently great, it may be necessary to apply a thin sheet of lead to the walls, if made of plasterboard, in order to provide the appropriate level of protection

If at all possible, the primary beam of the dental X-ray set should be directed towards an outside wall; it should *never* be directed against doors or doorways.

1.8   THE DENTAL X-RAY APPARATUS

The parameters controlling dental apparatus are given in section 33(1) of IRR 1985. When it has been assured that the administrative structure for radiation protection is in place, the most important practical requirement for maintaining satisfactory standards of radiation protection in the dental practice is to ensure that the X-ray apparatus is in good technical order and that the physical parameters of the radiation beam are correct. Consequently, all dental X-ray apparatus should be serviced regularly — at least every three years — by an engineer designated by the manufacturer.

However good, the X-ray apparatus — availability and proficiency of the service engineer is paramount.

In addition, it is obligatory that a full radiation and quality assurance survey is continuously carried out to prevent any inadvertent leakage or electrical fault. Fig 1.8.

As part of the assurance survey, the following parameters must be checked:

1. *Leakage*

Apart from the useful or primary beam, an X-ray tube produces radiation in all directions — principally around the primary beam, as the anode itself significantly attenuates radiation emitted in the direction of the electron beam. To prevent this radiation escaping through anything except the window of the X-ray tube head, from which the primary beam emerges, the lining of the tube casing must be radio-opaque.

2. *Filtration of the X-ray beam*

The dental X-ray tube head (Fig. 1.8) must have a filter fitted it to remove the soft or less penetrating components of the beam, which do not contribute to the formation of the radiographic image, but are absorbed into the superficial layers of tissue — an unnecessary radiation dose to the skin. The filter is one of the most effective ways of reducing skin dosage.

The filter should be fixed at the exit window of the tube head. The requirements for the filter thickness depend upon the operating voltage of the X-ray set:

- for voltages up to 70 kV peak [kVp], the filtration should be equivalent to 1.5 mm of aluminium
- for voltages above 70 kV, the filtration should be equivalent to 2.5 mm of aluminium, of which 1.5 mm must be fixed.

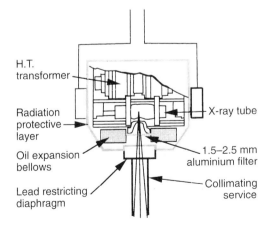

Fig. 1.8 Diagram of the tube head used for low-output dental apparatus.

3. *Collimation of the radiation beam*

Collimating devices must be used with dental equipment. They serve three purposes:

(a) They confine the X-ray beam to a small defined area, minimizing the risk of the irradiation of tissues outside the field of diagnostic interest. This confinement is initially achieved by the diaphragm — an integral part of the collimating device. The beam size is determined by the central aperture in the lead of which the diaphragm is made. The diameter of the X-ray beam at the surface of the skin must not exceed 6 cm (a measurement likely to be reduced in the new IRP regulations).

(b) To provide a standard anode–film distance

For operating potentials above 60 kV, the anode–skin distance must not be less than 20 cm. The longer the anode–skin distance, the more parallel the X-ray beam. This may necessitate a higher kilovoltage which will, within limits, reduce the radiation skin dose.

Modern apparatus employs more efficient multi-pulse techno-logy which gives a more constant beam of X-rays than the single-pulse system and, therefore allows the exposure time (mAs) to be reduced. Another development in modern dental apparatus is the position of the X-ray tube within the tube head (see Figure 4.10 page 66). This new technology allows for a longer anode–skin dose, as suggested in the 1994 Guidelines (NRPB 1994c).

(c) They allow a table of standardized exposure factors to be drawn up using fixed anode–film distances.

Types of collimating devices (Fig. 1.9)

1. *Circular or rectangular lead collimators*

These may incorporate film holders to give a very clearly defined area of irradiation. This will be of particular advantage in paralleling intra-oral techniques and general bitewing views.

The 1994 Guidelines (NRPB 1994c) recommend the use of rectangular collimators and, with appropriate training and judgement, this should be encouraged. See Figure 4.12a Figure 4.13.

2. *Cylindrical, 'open-ended' type cone*

These are often made of glass or plastic, to indicate the physical size of the field, with an interior metal cylinder. Whilst still in use, new apparatus incorporates a complete metal collimator.

3. *The old 'pointer' cone*

These are now illegal because of their lack of a clear-cut field of irradiation, with consequent increase of skin dosage. Particularly un-

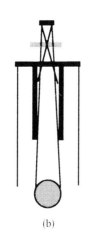 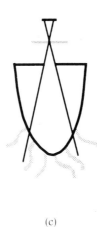

(a)   (b)   (c)

Fig. 1.9 Collimating devices limit the field of radiation. The complete metal collimator (a) superceded those with an internal metal cylinder that could produce a sharply defined field. The closed plastic device (c) acted as a source of scattered radiation and is now illegal.

acceptable was the fact that they employed such low, 'soft' kilo-voltages. Old apparatus using 'pointer cones' are not acceptable as they do not limit their X-ray beams to the required field of irradiation. See Fig. 2.9.

Operation and installation

The 1994 Guidelines (NRPB 1994c) discourage the use of apparatus with operating potentials below 60 kV. X-ray apparatus which is more than twenty years old must be given special attention.

When new dental apparatus is installed in a dental practice, it is the responsibility of the installer to ensure that it conforms to IRR 1985. Nevertheless, it would be sensible for the dental practitioner to check that this is the case.

The radiation protection supervisor has the responsibility, when new apparatus is installed, to hold the following specifications:

- name of manufacturer
- model number
- serial number
- year of manufacture
- year of installation.

Key points

1. Service equipment at least every 3 years
2. Leakage and electrical safety to be regularly checked
3. Filtration—1.5 mm A1 equivalent up to 70 kV — 2.5 mm A1 equivalent for 70 kV and over
4. Collimation of X-ray beam—to restrict field of radiation
5. X-ray beam at skin surface—6 cm maximum, likely to be reduced
6. Constant anode–film distance
7. Exposure factors, standardize
8. Operating potential not below 50 kV

1.9   DENTAL MONITORING SERVICES

Most local general hospitals offer a monitoring service through their medical physics departments. The National Radiological Protection

Board also offers a comprehensive radiation protection service for the dental profession. It is a postal service that extends over a period of 12 months with an option for annual renewal. For further information, write to: **The National Radiological Protection Board, Northern Centre, Hospital Lane, Cookridge, LEEDS, LS16 6RW. Tel. no. 0113 230 0232**

Either service provides:

(1) a set of outline local rules and an information package to assist in meeting legislative requirements;

(2) a technical assessment, by postal cassette, of each X-ray set in the practice;

(3) an assessment, based on a questionnaire, of the radiographic procedures in use;

(4) a practical check on the film processing facilities in use in the practice;

(5) a detailed report, giving recommendations, concerning equipment and procedures in relation to the relevant statutory requirements;

(6) advice and essential assistance with respect to any incident arising out of an equipment, malfunction or defect, as defined in Regulation 33 (2) of IRR 1985.

REFERENCES AND FURTHER READING

ICRP. (1977). *Annals of the ICRP*, **Vol. 1, No. 3**.

ICRP. (1991). *Annals of the ICRP*, **Vol. 21, Nos. 1–3**.

NRPB. (1995) *Radiation at Work: dental radiography*. NRPB, Didcat.

NRPB (1994*a*). *Radiation doses: maps and magnitudes*. NRPB, Didcat.

NRPB (1994*b*). *Radiation Protection Standards*. NRPB, Didcat.

NRPB. (1994*c*). *Guidelines on radiology standards for primary dental care*. NRPB, Didcat.

WALL. (1996). *Dosimetry and radiation protection explained: SYNERGY*.

NRPB. (1993). *Board statement on diagnostic medical exposures to ionising radiation during pregnancy: IRCP 26*. NRPB, Didcat.

ICRP. (1985). *Approved Code of Practice. The protection of persons against ionising radiation arising from any Work Activity. The Ionising Radiation Regulations*. HMSO, London.

DHSS. (1988). *Radiological protection in dental practice*. DHSS, London.

NRPB. (1990). *Living with radiation*. HMSO, London.

BMA. (1987). *The BMA Guide To Living With Risk*. John Wiley and Sons.

Dendy, P.B. and Heaton, B. (1987). *Physics for Radiologist*. Blackwell Scientific, Oxford.

Smith, N.J.D. (1988). *Dental Radiography* (2nd edn). Blackwell Scientific, Oxford.

Clarke, R.H. *Managing Radiation Risks.* (1997). Journal of the Royal Society of Medicine, **90**, Part 2, 88–92.

Horner, K. (1994). Radiation protection in dental radiology. *Br. J. Radiol.*, **67**, 803, pp.1041–9.

Haring, J.I., Lind, L.J. (1996). *Dental radiography: Principles and techniques.* W.B. Saunders & Co.

2 Factors affecting the radiograph image

2.1 THE LATENT IMAGE

X-rays, as part of the electromagnetic spectrum, have a similar effect on photographic film as light. Therefore, the image receptor can be a photosensitive emulsion formed of silver bromide crystals suspended in gelatin. The radiographic film has much in common with conventional photographic film. The effect of transmitted radiation upon the sensitive X-ray film will be the ionization of silver bromide crystals. This results in a specific pattern of silver ions within the emulsion which constitutes the latent image. The latent image is converted into a visible record by a series of chemical actions known as processing.

X-rays can also be utilized to convert X-ray photons into electrical signals. These can then be encoded into a digital record and displayed on a screen — now commonplace with computerised tomography. With this technique, it is now possible to place the phosphorbased sensor intra-orally, and transfer this computer-formed latent image directly on to a visual display unit. By incorporating a printer into the system, a hard copy image can then be obtained.

Before considering the details of these transformations, it is important to discover what factors affect the quality of the latent image. No amount of further chemical processing will improve the resulting image on the film, to provide information for clinical diagnosis. Digitizing systems do have the facility to enhance and manipulate the image. Nevertheless, the quality of the initial image will still be the limiting factor.

2.2 THE X-RAY BEAM

The quantity and quality of the radiation emitted from the X-ray tube head is dependent upon the milliamperage (mA) and the kilovoltage (kV). In dental X-ray apparatus it is necessary that the tube head should be easy to manoeure. This places a limit on the intensity or the milliamperage of the X-ray tube, and most apparatus operate at between 7 and 15 mA.

The quality of the X-ray beam is dependent upon the applied tube potential or kilovoltage. The high energy, short wavelength X-rays operating at higher voltages have greater penetrating power. In dental radiography, apparatus can operate at between 50 and 90 kVp With current knowledge of skin dosage at low kilovoltage — reinforced in legislation by the Ionizing Radiation Regulation (IRR) 1988 — and with the 1994. Guidelines on Radiology Standards for Primary Dental Care, it is hoped that apparatus operating below 60 kV will become a rarity. Nowadays' more apparatus is being manufactured at higher kilovoltages, that is 65–75 kVp.

Most dental X-ray sets have a fixed output, that is, the milliamperage and kilovoltage are preset. In a few, the kilovoltage is variable.

2.3   EXPOSURE FACTORS

The radiation exposure can be varied by changing the quantity and quality of the X-ray beam. It is important that these factors should be correctly assessed to produce dental radiographs of the highest possible diagnostic value. The required radiation exposure to the X-ray film depends upon:

- density of the object
- quality or penetrating power of the X-ray beam
- quantity of the X-ray beam
- sensitivity of the receptor — film or sensor
- anode–film distance
- field of irradiation.

2.3.1   Density of the object

The greater the density of the object, the greater will be the absorption of X-rays, and so less radiation will penetrate to reach the radiographic film or sensor. This will result in less blackening on the image. In intra-oral radiography, the range of densities within the object — the tooth and supporting bony structure — will be small.

More radiation will be absorbed in the upper molar region due to adjacent and overlying structures, therefore more radiation will be required.

2.3.2   Quality or penetrating power of the X-ray beam

The kilovoltage controls the penetrating power of the X-ray beam. In intra-oral radiography, where a variable kilovoltage is available, this can be utilized to increase the kVp for areas of greater density and to lower it when less dense, as in edentulous areas. It may also be lowered in an area where increased contrast is required, for example, to demonstrate a root canal. The ability to highlight the root canal, is one instance of the great value of the digitized image.

Lower kilovoltages will result in more clearly defined differences in penetration. The lower energy of the X-ray beam effectively means that this is more readily absorbed. So, with the tooth, low kilovoltages will be absorbed by the dentine and enamel, sometimes without differentiation, but will penetrate the root canal. In other words, the result is a sharper more 'black and white' image, with apparently more detail However, this is only the case within a limited range of densities.

In comparison, high kilovoltages allow more structures to be recorded, as the beam will have an increased sensitivity to the differences in densities. The resultant film has shades of grey and appears 'flatter', with less contrast — but with careful perception, more detail is in fact revealed.

When purchasing dental X-ray apparatus, it is important to consider the usefulness of lower and higher kilovoltages, balancing one against the other (Fig. 2.1).

Variations of kilovoltage are also controlled by legislation. IRR 1985 specifies requirements for the filtration and collimation of dental apparatus. These factors affect the quality of the X-ray beam — helping to reduce scatter and so prevent degradation of the image. The statutory obligations include:

1. There must be 1.5 mm of aluminium filtration for all dental tube voltages up to and including 70 kV, and 2.5 mm for voltages above 70 kV.

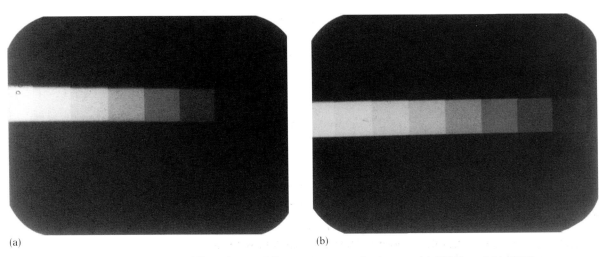

(a)   (b)

Fig. 2.1   Small step wedge on periapical films, showing differences in penetration between (a) 50 kVp and (b) 70 kV.

2. The diaphragm at the tube head must limit the field of irradiation to no more than 6 cm. If a longer object–film distance is possible, additional collimation must be added.

3. Apparatus operating above 60 kVp must have an anode–object distance of 20 cm.

4. If the longer anode–film distance of 40 cm is required, then the collimation must be appropriate to limit the field of radiation.

Examples of apparatus operating at differing kilovoltages, in use in the UK, are:

1. *Philips Gendex Oralix 65 65 kVp, 7.5 mA*
This apparatus gives a choice of timers, either dental symbols or time selection, and of collimator, for either 20 or 30 cm (Fig. 2.2 (a)).

2. *Belmont Belray 60 and 70 kVp 10 mA*

This apparatus gives the kilovoltage choice between 60 kV and 70 kV. This is important as there is also a choice of collimation between 20 cms or 35 cms.

It has constant potential technology which enables the exposure time to be cut by at least a third and consequently the radiation dosage is lessened.

• This apparatus has an exposure times, giving symbols not only for the teeth but also for the size of the patient and the speed of the film, which can include the digital image.

The exposure factors can also be pre-selected for either the 20 cm or the 35 cn anode-film distance.

• Today technology has evolved so that the X-ray tube can be positioned at the far end of the tube-head. This can allow a longer anode-film distance but with a conventional length collimating device. See Chapter 4 fig 4.9, p. 65.

3. *Schick (Keystone) Discovery DC 60 or 70 kVp 10 mA 35 cm FFD*

• S.S. White were one of the first manufacturers to place the X-ray tube at the rear of the tube-head behind the transformer giving this effective longer anode-film distance. Keystone X-ray purchased the firm in the 1980's and have continued in this tradition. Their Intrex dental intra-oral apparatus was introduced in 1982. There is now a new model—Discovery which can operate at 60 or 70 kV.

This longer anode distance allows the intra-oral paralleling technique to be undertaken more efficiently with less magnification, see Chapter 4, fig. 10, p 66.

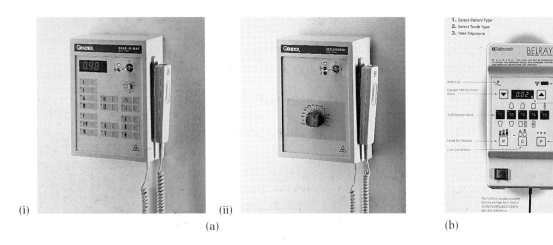

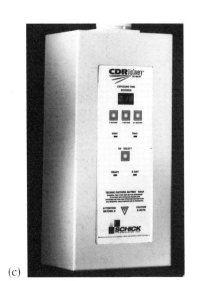

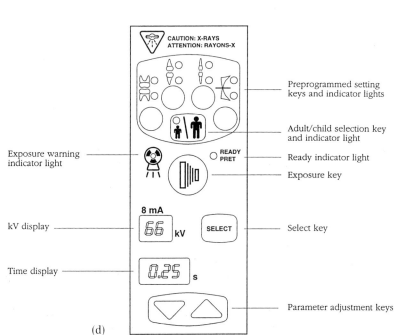

Fig. 2.2   (a) Philips Gendex Oralix 65S offers two timers: (i) Dens-o-mat, which gives dental symbol exposure choices; (ii) Secondent, which allows choices to be made according to a time selector. (b) Belmont's Belray uses dental symbol choices not only for anode distances and kilovoltages, but also to adjust exposure to include the density or size of the patient, and the speed of the film or the digital image. (c) Schick (Keystone) Discovery exposure timer, allowing a choice of 60 or 70 kV and exposure times which can be reduced to accommodate digital iamges. (d) Planmeca Prostyle Intra control panel allows for variations of kilovotages as well as milliampere times.

● The timer gives choice of of kilovoltage and can reduce the time to accommodate digital imaging Fig. 2.2c

4. *Planmeca Prostyle Intra 50–70 kV 8 mA*

This apparatus also has the X-ray-tube at the rear of the tube-head and can operate at either the 20 cm or 30 cms focal — film distance.

The longer anode-film distance can be achieved by the adition of extra collimation. This is attached to the existing collimation which is an integral part of the tube head. Rectangular field collimation can also be incorporated.

● Their hand held control panel uses symbols. It can be set for adult or child, and for the particular tooth. The exposures can be preset and then put into memory. There is a choice of kilovoltages in steps–50, 52, 55, 57, 60, 63, 66, 70. This allows for variations of density e.g. in edentulous areas and to highlight root canals during endodontics

5. *Siemens Heliodent DS 60 kV or 70 kV multipulse 7 mA*

The X-ray tube is at the rear of the X-ray tube head allowing a very neat 20 cm FFD unit.

This apparatus is also able to generate a high energy X-ray beam with a multipulse generator which has a stabler response to line voltage fluctuations. See Chapter 4, Fig. 4.10, p. 66.

● It can be used with chemical or digital imaging, by selecting the appropriate mode for the millampere exposure timing. The digital image needing only about a quarter of the exposure.

6. *IGE 1000* 50–100 kVp, 10 or 15 mA

For extra-oral dental radiography using dental apparatus, for example, oblique laterals, the same principles apply as for intra-oral radiography. However, as the area to be demonstrated is greater, the anode–object distance must be increased and the exposure factors calculated as indicated in the anode–film distance section.

In most dental panoramic tomographic apparatus, the milli-amperage and anode–object film distance are fixed, and the only variable is the kilovoltage. The IGE 1000, however, gives a full range of choices for both kilovoltage and milliamperage. So, the more dense the subject, the more penetrating can be the X-ray beam. When viewing the dental panoramic tomographic projection for children, the resultant radiograph appears bright and contrasting. For adults, the radiographs may appear less bright but there are gradients of density and, consequently, more detail within the focal trough is seen.

Key points

1. The latent image may be chemically produced-film or a computerised digital image-

2. X-ray beam —
   mAs – quantity – blackening of photographic or digital density dependant upon size of focal spot larger — increases thermal capacity but loss of detail
   kVp – quality – affects penetrating power and contrast; also produces some blackening.

When considering the choice of apparatus with consequent exposure factors there is something very important to bear in mind — the movement of the patient.

1. Higher kVs will lower the radiation dose and lower the exposure time, but will reduce the contrast.

2. Lower kVs will increase the radiation dose and lengthen the exposure time but enhance the contrast.

3. This is of particular significance with young children- time v quality.

A choice of kVs is the ideal.

2.3.3 Quantity of the X-ray beam

The quantity of the X-ray beam is governed to a large extent by the milliamperage and the exposure time, and is found by multiplying the tube current (in milliamperes (mA)) by the exposure time (in seconds). The result is expressed as milliampere seconds (mAs). With electronic timers, short exposure times can be accurately measured and, therefore, a higher milliamperage can be used to help compensate for movement, particularly when radiographing children. This is an important factor to bear in mind when considering the choice of apparatus.

1. The milliamperage will be limited by the size of the focal spot on the anode of the X-ray tube.

2. The larger the focal spot, the greater its thermal capacity and, therefore, the higher the permissible current — but this will lead to a loss of detail.

3. Thus, a compromise is reached between a focal spot of 0.5–1 mm and milliamperage between 7 and 15 mA.

A balance must be reached between the penetrating quality (kVp) of the X-ray beam and the quantity (mAs) in order to obtain optimum detail and contrast. If the kilovoltage is adjusted, remember to compensate the milliamperage to maintain adequate blackening of the film. An approximate guide is that by increasing the kVp by 10, the mAs can be reduced by half for the same anode–object distance:

1. Higher kVs will lower the radiation dose and shorten the exposure time, but will reduce the contrast.

2. Lower kVs will increase the radiation dose and lengthen the exposure time, but enhance the contrast.

The balance between time available and the resultant quality of image is of particular significance with young children. A choice of kilovoltages is the ideal (Fig. 2.3).

2.3.4 Sensitivity of the receptor

Intra-oral dental films are of different speeds. As with photographic film, the speed is controlled by the size of the crystals in the emulsion, slower film giving finer detail. Film speed relates to the amount of exposure needed to achieve a constant amount of blackening of the emulsion. It is recommended that the fastest films consistent with diagnostic interpretation should be used: Kodak Ultra speed film, group D; Ekta speed film, group E. (This latter film needs only half the radiation exposure, but there is some loss of detail.) (Fig. 2.4) (see also Fig. 1.7, p. 16)

The faster the film, the lower the margin of exposure time error. Contemporary technology is aiming to increase the speed of the film without appreciable lack of detail and contrast — but this has still to be achieved. Such an advance would allow the exposure time to be decreased, with consequent lowering of radiation dosage to the patient and, therefore, less risk to the operator.

Dental films

An X-ray film consists of a transparent, usually blue-tinted base, coated on both sides with a light-sensitive emulsion. A photographic emulsion is a suspension of minute silver bromide crystals in gelatin. The sensitivity of the emulsion depends upon the size of the crystals and the thickness of the emulsion which, on periapical and occlusal films, may be greater than the film used with intensifying screens. The practice of double coating the film reduces the exposure by half.

The intra-oral dental film is enclosed in a packet with a sheet of protective black paper on either side of it. A thin sheet of lead foil is placed on the side of the film remote from the tooth. The foil absorbs back scatter and so prevents fogging. Each film bears an embossed dot, the raised side of which indicates the side of the film that is placed towards the X-ray beam during exposure. The film, black paper, and foil are contained in a semi-stiff, moisture-proof, light-proof packet made from paper or plastic.

The position of the embossed dot is marked by an imprint on the outside of the packet. It is recommended that when the film is inserted into the patient's mouth, the embossed dot should be placed at the incisive margin of the tooth. This will prevent the superimposition of the film embossment at a vital area. It also helps to localize the position of the film in the patient's mouth, and so aid identification of the teeth from the radiograph.

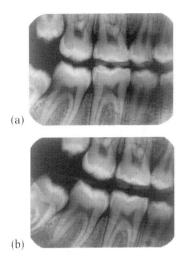
(a)

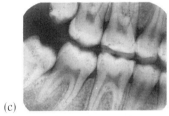
(b)

(c)

Fig. 2.3 Bitewing films demonstrating differences in exposures for different kilovoltages with a 10 milleamperage X-ray tube: (a) 50 kV, 1 second; (b) 60 kV, 0.6 seconds; (c) 70 kV, 0.3 seconds.

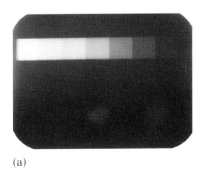
(a)

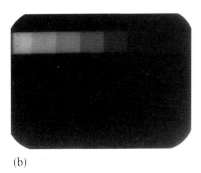
(b)

Fig. 2.4 Step wedge on periapical film of different speeds exposed to the same degree of radiation; (a) ultra speed; (b) Ekta.

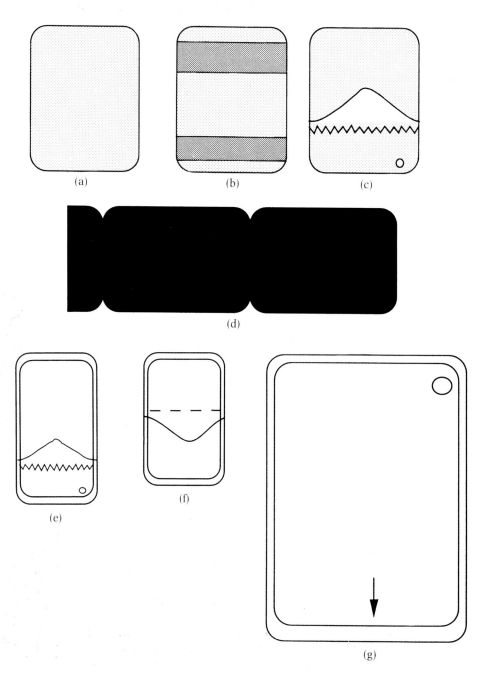

Fig. 2.5   Diagram of a dental film packet to show: (a) film; (b) lead foil backing of a 3.2 × 4.1 cm film; (c) outer packet; (d) interleaving paper. Also, actual sizes of (e) 2.2 × 4 cm film; (f) 2.2 × 3.5 cm film; (g) occlusal film.

Dental film is slower than a film-screen combination. It is also of a lower contrast, but this allows for greater latitude in the exposure range. Intra-oral films are supplied in the following sizes:

Periapical
3.2 × 4.1 cm
2.7 × 5.4 cm
2.2 × 4.0 cm
2.0 × 3.5 cm

Bitewings
3.2 × 4.1 cm
2.7 × 5.4 cm

Occlusal
5.7 × 7.6 cm
(Fig. 2.5)

The plastic-covered films are sealed in such a way that the edges and corners are very sharp. Great care should be taken to mould the corners, in particular, to minimize the discomfort to the patient. Do not *bend* the film corners as this will produce a dark line film fault. Plastic-covered films do bend easily, so it is important that the film is flat behind the tooth or teeth under examination (Fig. 2.6).

Intensifying screens

For extra-oral work, exposure can be reduced and contrast increased with the use of intensifying screens. These are used in pairs, one each side of the film.

Intensifying screens are housed in a cassette which is a light-tight, rigid container, to ensure contact between the film and screens. At the back of the cassette is a layer of lead foil to absorb back scatter. Some panoramic apparatus employ flexible screens (Fig. 2.7).

The original purpose of these screens was to improve the quality of the radiograph, but, today, the emphasis is on the reduction of radiation dosage. A reduction of the primary radiation beam passing through the object, before it reaches the film, will also reduce the amount of secondary, scattered radiation. This scattered radiation produces a grey fog over the primary image and, thus, degrades it by lessening the contrast.

An intensifying screen consists of a base coated with a phosphor material which emits light when irradiated with X-rays. The wavelength of this radiation is within the visible light spectrum, between ultraviolet and green. (Photographic emulsion is more sensitive to this than are X-rays.) The amount of light emitted from the phosphor screen is proportional to the amount of X-radiation passing through it.

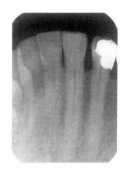

Fig. 2.6 Excessive curvature of film in the mouth.

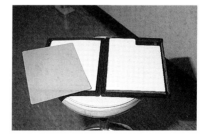

Fig. 2.7 Diagram of cassette housing intensifying screens to demonstrate: (a) rigid container with facility for white light naming device; (b) intensifying screens; (c) film.

The reduction in radiation possible will depend upon the type of phosphor. Calcium tungstate enables the dosage to be reduced by one-quarter for high definition screens and to one-tenth for fast screens.

The speed depends upon the crystal size, which is larger than that of the silver bromide in photographic emulsion, so loss of detail will occur in the resultant image.

In dental radiography, a balance must be achieved. It is useful to have a choice of screens depending on whether the information needed relates to bony detial or the mere presence of teeth.

Rare earth intensifying screens Technology is for ever advancing to create higher definition screens. Phosphors from the lanthanide series of earth elements, such as gadolinium and lanthanum, are now used in general radiography. They are more efficient in X-ray conversion and allow a further reduction in exposure, but with finer resolution. Although most screen phosphors emit blue or ultraviolet light, some rare earth screens emit green light. When using these screens, a film which is sensitive to green light (orthographic) must be used, together with brown or red dark-room safe lights. They are not very suitable for daylight processing.

Many of the original problems associated with rare earth screens have been solved, but this has made them more expensive. Rare earth intensifying screens allow orthodontists in general dental practice to take cephalometric lateral views of the facial bones with lower output apparatus.

Fast intensifying screens

It must be remembered that, as with faster films, the faster the intensifying screens, with consequent reduction of exposure factors, the smaller the margin of radiation exposure error. Before purchase, the general dental practitioner should consider carefully if the apparatus is sophisticated enough to cope with this reduction accurately, and also whether the processing facilities are adequate.

- Retaking radiographs due to over- or underexposure to X-rays will defeat the original purpose of the fast intensifying screens. With effective quality assurance, however, this difficulty may be overcome (*see* Chapter 16).

The computerized image

Modern technology allows a digitized image to be presented on a computer visual display monitor screen. The information contained in a conventional radiograph is analogue, that is, data represented in a continuous fashion. Digital information is in discrete units based upon the computer language of bytes and pixels. The great advantage of the digitized method is that only a relatively small amount of radiation is needed to create the latent image.

Key points

1. Speed is dependent upon size and type of crystals
2. Dental film — group D (ultra speed), Group D (Ekta)
3. Faster film, loss of detail
4. Intensifying screen
   — coated with phosphor
   — emit light when exposed to X-rays cut down radiation
   — some loss of detail
5. Rare earth screens, more efficient in X-ray conversion

However, direct digital dental radiology is now possible through two methods: one uses Charged-coupled devices (CCD); and the other uses photostimulable phosphor imaging plates. Both methods are suitable for the dental surgery, utilizing conventional personal computers (PCs).

1. *CCD*

An intra-oral sensor, analogous to a video camera, detects the X-rays and displays the image directly on the computer sceen. This system neccesitates the use of a cable which connects the sensor to the computer.

2. *Photostimulable phosphor imaging plates*

These are of a similar size as an intra-oral film and sensitive to X-rays, and can be positioned in the mouth in exactly the same way as the photographic dental film. After being exposed to the X-rays, the imaging plate is fed into a dedicated high-power laser 'processor', which incorporates a photo-multiplier to boost the signal, and visualizes the image on to the screen within 30 seconds.

The direct digital method: advantages

1. There is an instant exposure display and so patient involvement straightaway.
2. The image can be manipulated to help diagnosis, for example, to enhance the root canal or enlarge the periapical area.
3. There are fewer repeats due to exposure error.
4. Less ionizing radiation is required due to the image intensification.
5. The images are automatically stored and indexed, saving time and space.

The direct digital method: disadvantages

1. The results are improving all the time but are still not equal to the best photographic images.
2. Unfortunately, the sensor is not always as easy to position as photographic film:
    (a) It has a firm surface, which prevents inadvertent bending, but can be very uncomfortable for the patient and may lead to a lack of co-operation.
    (b) The sensor is thicker than dental film and may not fit the usual film holders. Some manufacturers have evolved their own holders, or adapted existing. ones.
    (c) The direct digital system has a 'free standing' sensor, but the CCD system has a cable attachment and often a thicker, cumbersome sensor.
3. The great danger of the digitized image for intra-oral radiography is that because the dose for the image is less than for conventional

Key points

The digital image

1. Less ionizing radiation
2. Instant exposure display
3. Image may be enhanced
4. Fewer exposure repeats

But

1. Image quality not equal to conventional radiograph
2. Not always easy to position the imaging plate
3. Uncomfortable for patient — hard and thick sensor

films, it is very tempting to repeat the procedure until one gets the best possible image.

4. Although the original image must always be stored — as specified in legislation in some countries — the manipulated image could give a misleading impression and have fraudulent implications (see Ch 7).

2.3.5   The anode–film distance

The anode–film distance is an important variable in calculating exposure factors. When using the short- or long-anode technique, the position of the collimating device should have a constant relationship to the skin surface. (See ch 4). This will help, too, in standardizing exposure factors or exposure times, as many low-output dental apparatus have fixed kilovoltage and milliamperage.

X-rays, like light rays, diverge along straight paths as they travel from their source, covering an increasingly larger area with ever-lessening intensity. This intensity (I) is inversely proportional to the square of the distance (d) from the source, that is, $I \times \frac{1}{d^2}$ This law is particularly relevant when calculating exposures for short- to long-anode intra-oral techniques.

Old mAs = old distance^2
New mAs = New distance^2
New mAs = new distance^2/old distance^2

If old mAs = 2.5
Old distance = 20 cm
New distance = 40 cm
Then new mAs = $40^2/20^2 \times 2.5$
= 1600/400 × 2.5
= 4 × 2.5
= 10 mAs

With milliamperage of 10 mA, Exposure time = 1 sec (Today, the exposure time would never be this long.)
The object density must remain constant.

2.3.6   Field of irradiation

The X-ray beam must be limited to the smallest coverage consistent with a good diagnostic film.

1. *Intra-oral radiographs:* the statutory code of Practice limits the field of radiation to a diameter of no more than 6 cm. (This may be

reduced in forthcoming legislation.) Preferably, a collimating device, incorporating the diaphragm, should be used. This will reduce scatter as well as protect the patient and operator. As recommended in the 1994 Guidelines (NRPB 1994), some dental apparatus now have rectangular collimation. Such apparatus is found mainly in dental hospitals, as the expertise necessary to avoid retakes seldom available in general dental practice. With a more extensive radiological and radiographic module within the dental curriculum it is hoped that this will change in the future.

2. Extra-oral dental radiography — oblique lateral projections: to include the greater area to be demonstrated, the anode–object distance must be increased. A balance should be reached between the exposure factor limitations of the apparatus, making it necessary to give long exposure times, and a shorter anode–object distance, where the enlargement factor will be present.

With higher kVp apparatus and a longer collimating device with a smaller diaphragm, a longer anode–object distance is an option. To cover an oblique lateral projection, the anode–object distance should be increased to 80 cm. This will cover a field of radiation with a diameter of 24 cm (inverse square law).

A summary of factors affecting the radiograph is given in Table 2.1 on page 38.

Key points

Exposure factors depend on

1. anode-film-distance standardisation if constant increase of distance — Xray beam looses intensity inversely proportionally to square of distance

    $$1 = \frac{x1}{d^2}$$

    If kV & mA are constant then 20 cm = Y mAs

    $$40 \ cm = \frac{40^2 \ x \ Y}{20^2}$$

2. Field of radiation intra-oral — 6 cm diameter extra-oral (oblique – lateral) usually 80 cm
3. Densisty of object

REFERENCES AND FURTHER READING

Waite, E. (1997) *Essentials of dental radiography* (2nd edn). Churchill Livingstone.

Champion Photochemistry and Photographic Technical Services. (1986). *Radiographic Processing*. Champion Photographic International Ltd, Brentwood, Essex.

Jenkins, D. (1980). *Radiographic photography and imaging processes*. MTP Press Ltd, Lancaster.

NRPB. (1994). *Guidelines on radiology standards for primary dental care.*.

Brocklebank, L (1996). *Dental radiology*. Oxford University Press.

Rohlin, M. and Hirschman, P.N. (1998). Designing an undergraduate curriculum in oral radiology is more than hours and content. *Editorial Dento-Maxillo Facial Radiology*, Vol. 27, No. 1, Jan 1998. Stockton.

Table 2.1   Factors affecting the radiographic image

Definition	Contrast	Limiting radiation hazards
Focal spot size Immobilization of patient Anode–object; object–film distance Speed of film Speed and type of in tensifying screens Diaphragm and collimating devices Grid	Kilovoltage Density of object Scattered radiation Chemical processing	Filtration Confining X-ray field Cutting radiation dosage by using fast films and intensifying screens Recommended anode–skin distance Raising kVp to lower skin dosage Digital imaging Lead apron for patient, if appropriate Distance of operator from primary and secondary beam

Temperature	Activity	Developing time
Density of object Film speed Intensifying screens Grid	Exposure factors Kilovoltage — kVp Milliamperage — mAs Time — mAs Movement	Anode–film distance Diaphragm size

	Digital image technology	
Improves with pixel matrix size	Digital options for Image enhancement may improve subjectively on the monitor with smaller visualization	

Careful radiographic techniques prevent retakes

3 Processing: techniques and specifications

3.1 INTRODUCTION

Processing is the collective name given to a series of operations carried out which effect chemical changes in the exposed film, thus making the latent image visible and permanent. The processing cycle may be carried out manually or automatically in or out of a specifically darkened room. The essential factor is for the exposed film to be protected from that part of the white light spectrum to which it is sensitive.

- It is important that the type of film or film screen combination, and the method of processing, are compatible.
- Generally, film for automatic processing may be processed manually, but not all films suitable for manual processing can be auto-processed.

When processing is undertaken outside a dark-room, the filtration from the white light is in the light-proof window (usually red) incorporated in the processor or an extension (Fig. 3.1). The light-proof compartment enables the operator to open the film packet or cassette

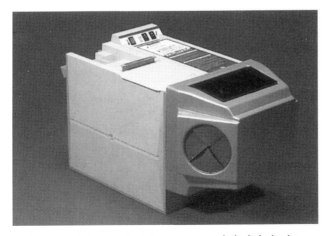

Fig. 3.1 Velopex automatic processor with daylight loader.

to feed the film into the processor, and is entered through a glove-like opening.

● Care must be taken not to allow the light to enter the processor and fog the film when removing the hands.

So, always make sure that the film is protected independently or is already fully within the developing tank. Another weakness in this system of light-proofing lies in the elasticity of the glove extension. It should be checked regularly and replaced when slack.

If space is available, much more satisfactory results are achieved with a proper dark-room. This is especially so when extra-oral views, employing the use of cassettes, are regularly taken.

Some of the light-proof compartments on day light processors allow for the cassette to be opened and the film fed into the processor, but few allow for the cassette to be repacked — an exception is the Durr XR 25 with a daylight attachment, DL 24 (Fig. 3.2).

Positioning of daylight processors, whether manual or automatic, is important. If placed near very bright lights, for example, sunlight, the filtration of the viewing window will not be adequate and fogging of the film will occur (see Ch. 16).

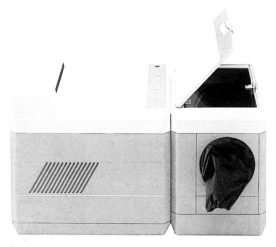

Fig. 3.2   Durr XR 25 processor with DL 24 extension in which cassettes can be reloaded.

3.2   THE DARK-ROOM

The dark-room must be light-proof in that all white light — artificial or daylight — has been excluded. It should be sited as near as possible to the operating radiographic room and be adequately protected against penetrating radiation. All doors, blinds and panels in a dark-room require to be fitted closely, to prevent any leakage of light into the room. It should be possible to lock the door during processing or put a warning light outside. In general lay out, a dark-room should be large enough to allow free movement. Specific factors to consider include:

1. There should be enough space for tanks and their containers, for manual processing. For automatic processing, there must be a horizontal area large enough to take the processor with access at both ends. The best situation for an automatic processor is through a wall, so that the dry films can be collected without disturbing the fresh input of film. Such a siting can also reduce the area necessary within the dark-room. However, modern automatic processor design does not facilitate this, since the film exits over the top of the processor, to reduce the size of the machine.

2. Adequate bench space is essential — either on the opposite side to a manual processing unit, or separated from it by an effective anti-splash shield. Splashes of any liquid on to a dry film will mark it and impair its diagnostic value. The dry bench should be approximately 100 cm high and 60 cm deep. It may incorporate cupboards for films and chemicals, although it is usually thought advisable not to keep these together, and for them to be stored outside the dark-room. A dark surface to the bench helps to show up films, when taken from a packet or cassette.

3. Ventilation is important, since in most cases the dark-room will be small and the chemical fumes are potentially hazardous.

●   The recommended ventilation rate is 12 air changes an hour.

4. It is undesirable to work in absolute darkness, and so safety lighting is used in dark-rooms. Safe lights are lamps fitted with filters which allow only those wavelengths to which the film is relatively insensitive to pass through — usually the red part of the light spectrum. Care must be taken to follow the maker's instructions in the use of the correct wattage bulbs and the distance from the working surface. Excessive exposure, even to a safe light, may cause fogging.

●   The usual recommendation is a 25 W pearl bulb which is placed 1.2 m from the bench top.

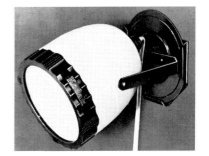

Fig. 3.3 Kodak Beehive safelamp. This can be fitted to a work-bench, shelf, or wall, or suspended from the ceiling. (Reproduced with kind permission of Kodak.)

Check regularly for cracks in the safe light filter as this can fog the films. Usually, two safe lights are desirable — one ceiling reflector over the dry bench and another on the wall to illuminate the processing tanks (Fig. 3.3). A white viewing lamp is useful for examining the radiographs while still wet, but fixed. With manual processing, it is

Key points

1. Light-tight room
2. Good ventilation — 12 air changes per hour
3. Cleanliness
4. Organisation of equipment
5. Proper safe lighting, with correct wattage of the bulb and no cracks in the filter
6. Thermometer — ideal processing temperature is 20 °C
7. Timer — to time films in the developer and fixer, correctly

important to rinse the X-ray holder in water before viewing the films as fixer drips, being acid, can damage the processing surround.

If there is any doubt about the reliability of the safe light illumination, it can be tested easily by opening a dental packet and placing the film on the dry bench, with a coin on top. If left for one minute and processed as usual, no outline of the coin should be seen. A more precise way to monitor safe lights is to place five small coins in a row on an occlusal film. Put a piece of cardboard over four of the coins. Leave this film on the bench for 50 seconds and at 10-second intervals reveal another coin. Visually, it is then possible to check if the safe light is too strong or too near the bench.

5. It is essential that the dark-room should be kept spotlessly clean because X-ray film is very sensitive to any form of contamination. Films should never be handled with wet or even damp fingers — finger-marks cannot be removed from processed films (see Ch. 16). The dental film packet should be held along its edges, between thumb and index finger, and the outer wrapping and lead packaging removed so that the freed film can be securely fixed in one of the dental clips, or fed into the processor.

6. Every piece of equipment demands a definite place in the dark-room and must be kept readily accessible when sought in safe light conditions, for example, film hangers on racks.

3.3   MANUAL PROCESSING: SPECIFIC REQUIREMENTS

1. The four processing tanks should be contained in a large porcelain or stainless steel sink, with a hot and cold water supply. It is as well to site the taps some distance above the tanks to allow free movement of the film hangers in and out of the tanks. Ideally, the processing tanks should be immersed in a thermostatically controlled water jacket (Fig. 3.4). The developer tank should have a lid to prevent fogging of the film, and to reduce both the level of fumes in the dark-room and also oxidation of the chemicals. The film is usually developed for 5 minutes at 20 °C, depending on the manufacturer's recommendations, but it is important that the temperature should be correct to ensure optimum developer activity.

2. When the films have been safely unwrapped they can be placed upon single clips or special hangers on which there are differing numbers of clips (Fig. 3.5). Care must be taken that the dental films are placed carefully on the hangers so that they do not overlap and all parts of the film are evenly exposed to chemical action (see

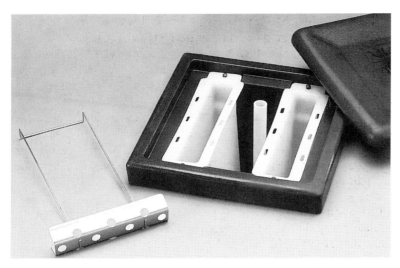

Fig. 3.4   Rinn processing tank with water jacket and cover.

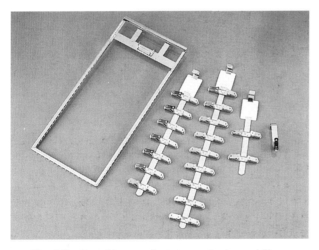

Fig. 3.5   Dental hangers for intra- and extra-oral films.

Ch. 16). When placing the hangers into the developer, they should be agitated slightly to release air bubbles and to keep the solution evenly distributed, thus ensuring consistent chemical activity. The developer in the tank should be stirred at least once a day before use, and every time it is topped up. The hangers must also be spaced carefully so they are not in contact with each other.

3. A thermometer and immersion heater are important items of auxiliary equipment. A timer is also necessary to standardize development time. Time and temperature are vital factors in processing and in establishing exposure factors and, consequently, quality assurance.

Key points

1. Development — 5 minutes at 20 °C; do not open the darkroom door
2. Rinse — to wash off developer
3. Fixing — for twice the time for films to clear
4. Wash — 10 minutes, in fresh running water
5. Drying — in dust-free atmosphere
6. Mount and correctly label the films
7. *Advantages*
   — Cheap to run
   — Cheap to install
   — Low maintenance
   — Easy to use

Disadvantages
   — Chemicals need changing frequently
   — Proper temperature control
   — Manual replenishment
   — Dark-room needed
   — Films to be dried manually

4. A rinse tank is needed to remove surface developer and thus stop further development of the film. The hanger and film should be held to drain above the developer tank to prevent excessive and expensive contamination, and then given a short dip in a rinse tank.

5. The film is then placed into fixer for about 10 minutes, and should not be exposed to white light until it has been there for at least two minutes. The fixing time is calculated as twice as long as it takes to clear the unexposed parts of the film (dissolve the unexposed silver bromide). Again, before washing the film, drain any excess fixer by holding it above the tank.

6. The film is washed in running water for 10–15 minutes, depending upon the water flow. If this is not possible, the water in the tank should be changed at frequent intervals to prevent contamination — as often as twice daily if the throughput is high, but at least once a day.

7. The film must be dried either in a drying cabinet or in a dust-free atmosphere, then labelled with the correct name and date.

3.4   AUTOMATIC PROCESSING: SPECIFIC REQUIREMENTS

Automatic processing involves the same stages as manual processing, with the exception of rinsing between the developer and fix. This stage is omitted because excess developer is either drained (Durr Periomatic) or squeezed (Durr XR 24, XR 25, Gendex Gxp) back into the developer tank during the processing cycle.

Most important is the fact that automatic processors are thermostatically controlled, with the developer used at a higher temperature to speed up its activity, for example, 30 seconds at 30 °C. The film then passes into the fixer, leaving this tank again through squeegee rollers to prevent carrying over chemicals into the wash tank. Finally, the film enters the drying process — usually heated air (Fig. 3.6).

The most efficient of the automatic processors have built-in replenishing tanks positioned under the processor which, automatically, or by pressing an action button, will refill the tanks with more chemicals as and when required. If the processor tanks are not at the correct activating temperature, or completely filled, the films will not be adequately processed.

There are many dental processors on the market. They vary in their degree of automation and sophistication, and consequent limitations. Two popular models are:

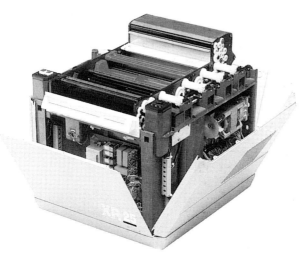

Fig. 3.6 Durr XR 25 automatic processor with roller system.

Durr Periomat (Fig. 3.7)

This is the simplest processor and an efficient apparatus, within its limitations. It takes periapical films and, with holders, will accept small periapical and occlusal films. It is usually operated under daylight conditions. When the films have been removed from their packets and inserted into position, they progress up and down grooves, in a snake-like path.

This processor is not thermostatically controlled, nor has it running water, so it is very important to change the washing water very

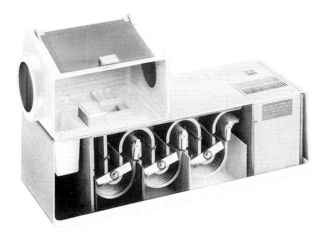

Fig. 3.7 Durr Periomat Processor with 8-channel film transport system with synchronized rotation arms.

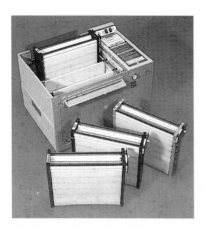

Fig. 3.8 Velopex automatic processor with webbing transport system.

Key points

1. Development, fixing, rinsing, and drying in one processor — thus, shorter processing times
2. Webbing and roller transport mechanisms take extra- and intra-oral films
3. Automatic replenishment available
4. Cleanliness essential
5. Regular quality assurance monitoring
6. *Advantages*
   — Dark-room not always needed
   — Usually temperature-controlled
   — Automatic replenishment available
   — Set processing time
   — Easier to standardize for quality control

   Disadvantages
   — Expensive to buy
   — Needs regular maintenance

frequently, keep the chemicals at the correct level, and check for temperature changes. The quality of the resulting image is, however, very good (always assuming the processor is looked after properly). This is probably because the processing time is about nine minutes, compared to most modern machines which have shorter cycles.

Velopex (Fig. 3.8)

This processor uses a system of plastic webbing to move the film forward. Sometimes, the films can have the pattern of the webbing on the image, which can detract from the quality. The Velopex does not automatically replenish the chemicals — only the water — but it is thermostatically controlled.

●   It cannot be stressed strongly enough that regular cleaning of processors is of the utmost importance.

In most automatic processors, the films travel by the use of rollers small enough to transport dental films. The timing of the complete processing cycle will be slower than in those processors designed just for extra-oral films — between 5 and 10 minutes, compared to 90 seconds. This is due to the thickness of the emulsion. Extra-oral film processors are not necessary in general dental practice, as the slow dental processors will also take extra-oral films up to the limit of their width, for example, Durr XR 24 or XR 25 (see Fig. 3.6). Both of these processors are automatically replenished and thermostatically controlled. They can be used in or out of the dark-room.

The Durr also has a rapid programme for endodontic use, allowing films to be viewed after three minutes instead of seven minutes. If these films are then needed for storage, they can be returned to the normal programme, for fixing and washing. Durr and Rinn produce 'chairside' processors which develop intra-oral radiographs in a short time using rapid processing chemicals. These are also suited for endodontic work, when a quick result is required (Figs 3.9 and 3.10).

All automatic processors need very special cleaning of the moving parts for successful maintenance — thorough soaking and wiping of the rollers, and cleaning with hot water and a sponge or soft brush. A toothbrush is useful for cleaning the cogs in the small Durr processor and the Velopex. In the Velopex, the static electricity (see Ch. 16) which can build up in the plastic webbing will be lessened with the use of fabric softener rinse. Abrasive surface cleaners should not be used, whilst recommended cleaning fluid can be obtained for occasional use, when necessary. It is always best to abide by the manufacturer's instructions.

All processing systems should be regularly monitored for quality assurance (*see* Chapter 16) as processing is a vital link in producing diagnostic radiographs.

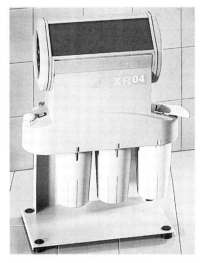

Fig. 3.9   Durr XR04 X-ray film developer.

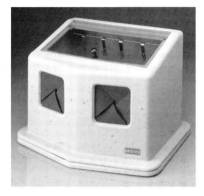

Fig. 3.10   Rinn 'chairside darkroom'.

3.5   SELF-DEVELOPING FILMS

Self-developing X-ray film comes in a plastic, flexible container which holds the processing chemicals in a compartment, away from the unexposed film. When the radiograph is ready to be processed, a

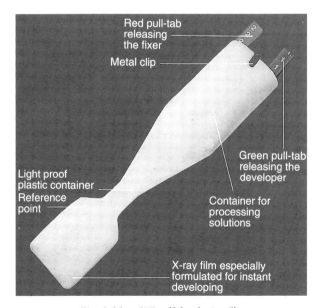

Fig. 3.11   GXR self-developing film.

green tab is withdrawn to release the developer into the sachet containing the film. This is manipulated for about 30 seconds, then the procedure is repeated with a red tab, to release the fixer. The solutions are discarded and the film is washed under running water and then dried (Fig. 3.11).

Advantages

- No dark-room required
- Time saving

Disadvantages

- Resulting image is not good quality
- Image does not last over time
- Procedure can be messy when discarding the chemicals
- Relatively expensive
- Film packet is flexible and difficult to position

3.6   THE CHEMICAL COMPONENTS OF THE PROCESSING CYCLE

3.6.1   Developer

Developer is the first chemical into which the film is immersed during the processing cycle and it is alkaline (pH 7+). Its purpose is to reduce the exposed areas of the film to metallic silver, rendering the latent image visible. Its efficiency depends upon how well it can distinguish between the exposed and unexposed silver halide. It comprises:

1. *Developing agents*

(a) Phenidone: this is a fast but low-contrast developing agent.
(b) Hydroquinone: this is a slow but high-contrast developing agent, the activity of which is closely allied to temperature.

Most developers are a combination of these two agents and are named PQ developers. Developer activity is dependent upon temperature and concentration of chemicals.

2. *Accelerator*: potassium carbonate is an essential element of developer, being an alkali component that will enhance the activity of hydroquinone.

3. *Restrainer*: benzotriazole is a chemical that retards the action of the developing agents on the unexposed areas of the film.

4. *Hardener*: glutaraldehyde hardens emulsion and prevents softening and damage during automatic processing. However, glutaraldehyde

is hazardous and certain manufacturers no longer use it, or have reduced its levels in their developer.

5. *Preservative*: sodium or potassium sulphite reduces excessive oxidation of the developing agents, but cannot eliminate it. If the lid is left off the developing tank, the preservative will be used up rapidly.

6. *Fungicide*: prevents the growth of bacteria during storage and use.

7. *Buffer*: hydrogen ions are a by-product of the development process. Consequent changes in the pH would influence the activity of the developer, so a buffering system is used to maintain the pH within specific limits that is, ± 0.05 pH units.

8 *Solvent*: water.

3.6.2   Rinse

As already stated, rinsing is only necessary in manual processing to wash off excess developer.

3.6.3   Replenisher

Replenisher has similar components to developer, but in a different ratio. There is no restrainer, as the process of reducing the silver bromide will gradually increase the bromide content of the developing solution. Also, the percentage of preservative is increased — so it is very important to keep a lid on the replenisher tank.

With manual processing and non-replenishing automatic processors, replenisher is not essential — topping up with developing solution is sufficient.

With automatically replenished processors, replenisher prolongs the life of the developer. The amount required depends upon the size of the tanks. Most automatic processors in common usage in dental practices and dental radiology departments do not use developing tanks with a capacity of more than 7.5 litres, and many tanks are considerably smaller. Under these circumstances, a complete change of developing solution is often an easy option and an advantage. At the same time, the rollers and tanks can be thoroughly and regularly cleaned to prevent the growth of bacteria.

3.6.4   Fixer

The developing solution removes the bromide from the exposed silver bromide crystals without substantially affecting the underexposed crystals. The undeveloped silver bromide gives the film a dense opalescent appearance and, if exposed to light in this state, the film will darken slowly, obscuring the image. Fixer renders the unexposed silver bromide soluble, so that it can be dissolved out of the emulsion and into the fixer solution, thus making the image permanent. It has a pH of less than 7 and so is acidic. It comprises:

1. *Fixing agent*: ammonium thiosulphate removes silver bromide without adverse effects on the film.

2. *Acid*: acetic acid ensures the pH of the solution and will counteract any of the developer which might be carried over into the fixer.

3. *Preservative*: sodium metabisulphate helps to prevent decomposition of the fixing agent.

4. *Hardener*: aluminium chloride or sulphite is used. Since hardening of the emulsion takes longer than the removal of unexposed silver halides, more time is required for the film to fix properly than for it to clear — approximately twice as much.

Silver test papers can be obtained to measure the amount of silver dissolved from the unexposed silver bromide present in the solution. This can reach a level where the fixing bath is no longer efficient (the pH has fallen) and the films do not come out clear but have a greenish yellow tint. This is know as dichroic fog. The lowering of acidity in the fixer allows development to continue for a short time, and a silver colloid to form over the surface of the film. Lack of rinsing in manual processing or contamination of the fixer with developer also produces this fogging. The chemical baths must then be replaced. The silver test papers provide a measurement for comparison with a density graduation scale. The accepted level of silver to render the fixing bath exhausted is about 6 g/h. For small tanks, it is practical to change the fixer when it takes twice as long for the films to clear as in fresh solution.

5. *Solvent*: water.

3.6.5   Washing

It is necessary to wash out the fixer products from within and on the surface of the emulsion. These cause image fading and discoloration on storage. In manual processing, about 15 minutes washing in running water is required. This time can be decreased by agitation and by increasing the temperature of the heater. Obviously, it must be still within the limits that ensure hardener efficiency. Wash tanks in automatic processors should be emptied at night.

3.6.6   Drying

In manual processing, after draining off the excess water, the films should be placed in a drying cabinet or hung up in a well-ventilated and dust-free place. Care must be taken that the wet emulsion is not touched or damaged in any way. In particular, films should not be splashed with water during drying, as this will produce spots which cannot be removed. The rate at which water can be removed from the emulsion surface depends greatly upon the air temperature and its humidity level. The higher the former and the lower the latter, then the faster, within limits, will the film be dried.

3.7   PREPARATION OF PROCESSING CHEMICALS

It must be remembered that processing chemicals, particularly when concentrated, are harmful if mishandled. When preparing the chemical baths avoid contact with the skin and eyes, and wear protective clothing and rubber gloves. Pour the chemicals slowly, as the instructions suggest. The preparation should be in a well-ventilated room to prevent inhalation, using separate utensils for the developer and fixer to avoid contamination. Although there is considerable latitude in the use of some developers, care should be taken if automatic processing developers are used for manual processing. The hardener incorporated in these developers for high temperatures is harmful to the hands.

Key points

1. Keep chemicals away from children and animals
2. Read the manufacturer's instructions before preparing chemicals
3. Use protective gloves, aprons, and eye-shields when preparing chemicals and cleaning tanks
4. Good ventilation is essential
5. Keep all equipment and work areas clean to avoid contamination

3.7.1   Silver recovery

In multiple practices, particularly where cephalometric films and panoramic views are taken, silver recovery should be considered. Silver is an expensive commodity and a diminishing world resource. X-ray film contains silver bromide but only part of the silver remains in the resultant radiograph, the remainder passing into the fixing solution. It is possible to recover 98 per cent of silver from a waste fixer, and it is estimated that from 1 sq m of film, 5 g of silver is potentially recoverable. The following old methods of silver recovery are being phased out in many imaging departments:

- electrolysis for example, PSR Silver King
- metallic replacement, for example, steel wool recovery units.

In most X-ray departments, the fixer is collected by special firms which pay according to volume. However, this means that there must be storage space for the containers which can pose problems.

It is recommended that if the exhausted fixer is just discarded, it should be diluted before disposal into the water drainage system, otherwise contamination can occur and local water authority rules may be contravened. Old films are also a source of silver recovery.

3.8   XERORADIOGRAPHY

Xeroradiography is a diagnostic system which allows images to be recorded using the xerographic copying process. This technique has the ability to produce images of both soft and hard tissues, and gained popularity in the 1960s with its application to mammography. It was later applied by orthodontists to lateral cephalometry. Much experimental work was carried out in the 1970s on using this technique for intra-oral radiography, concluding that xeroradiographic images were diagnostically superior to conventional film in detecting tooth, bone, and soft tissue changes, principally because of the greater exposure latitude and the unique property of edge enhancement. The technique has been applied to periodontics and to the detection of small caries lesions.

In xeroradiography, the silver halide emulsion used in conventional radiography is replaced by an aluminium plate backing which carries a thin plate of selenium, to which a uniform positive charge is applied. When exposed to X-rays, the plate is discharged in proportion to the degree of radiation penetrating through the object to be recorded. Subsequently, this latent image is made visible by passing it through a solution containing toner particles which are attracted to the selenium plate. These are transferred to a clear tape with white backing.

The disadvantage of xeroradiography is that the small intra-oral plate is hard and uncomfortable in the mouth, and the developing process is somewhat temperamental. Nevertheless, the images produced give excellent diagnostic information (Fig. 3.12) and can best be utilized in specialist, well-monitored units.

(a)

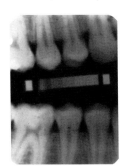

(b)

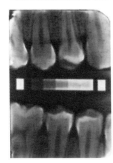

Fig. 3.12   Bitewing radiographs of right premolar and first molar region processed by (a) chemical action and (b) xerographic method.

3.9   MOUNTING RADIOGRAPHS

After drying, the radiographs should be mounted in such a way that they can be studied under proper illumination. Loose radiographs can be easily lost or damaged, and all films should be mounted and marked with the patient's name and a relevant date — not only for viewing and identification but also for record purposes.

Many suitable mounts are available to hold dental radiographs. They are made of light card or plastic, with openings into which the radiographs slide and where they are securely held. Another safe and simple method of mounting is to staple radiographs on to a sheet of thin, flexible, translucent acetate material. A label is firmly attached, with the patient's name and date of X-ray written on it. The acetate sheeting is then cut to the appropriate size.

Before the films are affixed, they should be arranged in their correct order from right to left, upper and lower jaw, as though one were looking into the mouth of the patient. This is done simply if the raised side of the embossed dot is towards the examiner. The only exception to this rule is in the case of the lower, true occlusal films, which are turned with the concave surface upwards so that the line of the mandible is again as if looking into the patient's mouth.

When using cassette films, the letters 'R' and 'L' are placed to identify which side of the patient is which. The rule on correct order still applies and, the letters having been placed so that the view of the patient is from the front, the appropriate side can be fixed. With oblique lateral extra-oral films, there is no unanimity as to viewing, but if comparing them with intra-oral films, it is again easier to place the letters and the details of identification as if facing the patient.

The radiographs should be viewed on a viewing box (Fig. 3.13) which has uniform lighting, in a room in which the lighting is subdued. A magnifying glass is useful.

Key points

1. Films should be mounted in the correct order, as if looking at the patient
2. The raised dot should be towards the examiner
3. The correct name, date, and identification number must be clearly marked on the mounting material

---

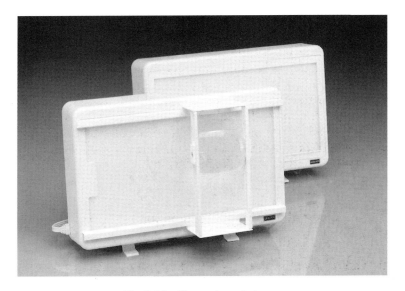

Fig. 3.13　Rinn universal viewer.

3.10   CONCLUSION

It is important that correct and accurate processing is achieved, so that high-quality radiographs of good density and contrast are produced. Failure to do this may result in having to repeat radiographs, thus increasing the radiation dose to the patient. All films must be of good diagnostic value, whilst the radiation dose to the patient is kept as low as reasonably achievable.

REFERENCES AND FURTHER READING

Jenkins, D. (1980). *Radiographic photography and imaging processes*. MTP Press Ltd, Lancaster.

Jeromin, L.S., Geddes, G.F., White, S.C., and Gratt, B.M. (1980). Xeroradiography for intra-oral dental radiography. *Oral Surgery, Oral Medicine, Oral Pathology*, **49**, 173–83.

Wilson, N.H.F. and Grant, A.A. (1986). A clinical trial of dental xeroradiography. *British Dental Journal*, **161**, 327–35.

4 Intra-oral radiography: I

4.1 INTRODUCTION

Intra-oral radiography is a technique which uses small dental films placed in the mouth to obtain an image of all or part of the teeth, alveolar margins, and supporting bone. Sometimes, the bone beyond the apex needs to be included, for example, to demonstrate unerupted teeth or more extensive apical pathology.

The horseshoe configuration of the dental arches means that only one, two, or at most, three teeth can be projected on to a film at one time. So, many films will be necessary to include the complete dentition. However, the advent of panoramic dental tomography, in addition to the other established extra-oral technique — oblique laterals — makes it possible to obtain one overall view, on which areas of interest can be pinpointed. Thus, intra-oral radiographs can be kept to a minimum and ionizing radiation kept 'as low as reasonably achievable' (see p. 18). Nevertheless, accurate intra-oral radiographic views give an undistorted image, with much greater detail than any extra-oral projection.

4.2 ANODE–OBJECT DISTANCE

The ideal radiographic situation is when the object and the film are parallel and in close proximity, and a parallel X-ray beam is directed at right angles to them. This will project the perfect image with no enlargement or distortion. To obtain *an almost* parallel X-ray beam, the anode–object distance should be 1.8 m. This anode–object distance is utilized in orthodontic practice, with a little compromise, when covering the large area necessary to produce a lateral projection of the facial bones with minimal enlargement.

The centre of the X-ray beam will always contain parallel rays, but with shorter anode–object distances these may not extend to cover the complete field of irradiation. For intra-oral radiographic techniques, with a maximum field of irradiation of 6 cm diameter at the

Key points

Ideal radiograph
1. Tooth and film parallel
2. X-ray beam at 90° to both
   bitewings
   — parallel film technique
3. BUT, not always
   anatomically possible

skin surface, an anode–object distance of 40 cm will give *an almost parallel beam*.

The option of an apparatus with a 40 cm anode–object distance has become important within dental hospital X-ray departments so that the best possible image can be produced. In general practice, the Ionising Radiation Regulations (IRR) 1985 and the 1994 Guidelines on Radiology Standards for Primary Dental Care can be expected to necessitate the replacement of some of the very old, low-output dental apparatus by those operating above 60 kVp which require an anode–object distance of 20 cm rather than 10 cm. This longer distance allows greater choice in intra-oral perapical techniques, as well as reducing radiation dosage to the skin.

4.3   PATIENT POSITION

Historically, dentistry was practised in an upright dental chair. Consequently, the dentist took the radiograph in that position. Today, with low-level dentistry and modern equipment, many practitioners wish to take their radiographs in this position. It is obviously a time-saving and more convenient position X-ray apparatus is evolving that offers much more flexibility, a longer reach, and smaller and lighter tube heads. All that is necessary to work in the horizontal plane is for the X-ray tube head to be so positioned that it is readily accessible. Hopefully, manufacturers will make it easier for the tube head to be operated in the horizontal, working position by including a facility to adjust the angles on the dial round the tube head accordingly.

However, at the present time, many dentists still take their dental radiographs with the patient sitting upright — except perhaps for endodontic control films.

It can be claimed that as the dentist has to stand two metres away before exposing the films, the patient may as well be moved into the more familiar vertical radiographic position.

One advantage of this position is that landmarks can be easily located in relation to the X-ray tube, which can rotate around the patient, providing intra-oral radiographs from both sides of the head.

The vertical position is the position of preference for dental hospital X-ray departments, and Group practices where there is a separate X-ray room which may also include panoramic apparatus. (It is essential, under these cicumstances, that safeguards are set up to ensure that only one apparatus can be operated at a time.)

The horizontal, working position is mainly for the dentist in practice, which includes the undergraduate learning to apply the same standard intra-oral radiographic techniques in both positions (Fig. 4.1).

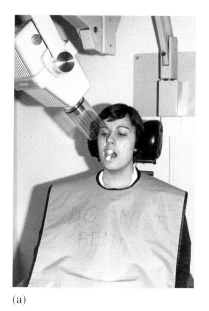
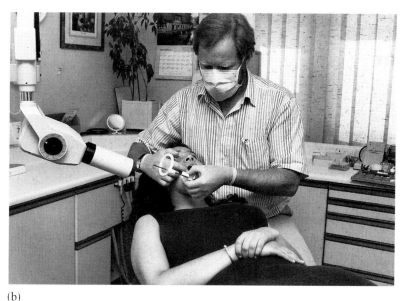

(a)   (b)

Fig. 4.1   (a) Patient seated with film and holder for bisecting angle periapical technique; (b) patient in dental working position ready for paralleling periapical technique.

The vertical and horizontal planes for stabilizing the head are adjusted through 90° in the horizontal, working position and, where necessary, the head is rotated as well as the tube.

The angle of the X-ray beam, in relationship to the tooth and occlusal plane, is still of prime importance in the horizontal, working position. Otherwise, there is no baseline for assessing those inadvertent errors or unexpected findings that necessitate further films.

4.4   BITEWING RADIOGRAPHY

- Where the object and film are parallel and in close proximity, as in bitewing radiography, there is little advantage in the extra long anode–object distance. Bitewing radiography is the name given to the lateral projection of the crowns of teeth in both the upper and the lower jaws, together on one film, with the interdental spaces also demonstrated.

- Bitewing radiography is very important in dentistry. Many dentists take control bitewings at regular intervals, depending upon the patients clinical history relating to the incidence of caries. They disclose:

(1) the extent of caries — suspected and unsuspected — and may reveal the presence of recurrent caries under restoration;

(2) the relationship between a prepared cavity and the pulp chamber, showing an overhanging edge of a restoration;

(3) information for the diagnosis of periodontal disease (see Fig. 4.6).

As only the crowns and periodontal margins are to be examined, both maxilliary and mandibular teeth can be projected on the same film. There must be some means of immobilizing the film behind the crowns. The most usual method is the commercially produced 'bitewing' film, with the addition of a tab for the patient to bite upon. Bitewing films are available in standard dental film sizes — 3.2 × 4.1 cm and 2.7 × 5.4 cm.

The latter size should be used sparely and carefully. Unless the size of the patient's mouth warrants the use of this film, the extra length is often wasted behind the crowns of the last molar tooth, causing discomfort. It may be used legitimately to show the presence of third molars, as well as the interproximal spaces.

Tabs may be obtained separately and stuck on to standard dental films, horizontally — or vertically for anterior spaces. 2.2 × 3.5 cm film may also be used vertically for a specific space, or horizontally in paedodontics.

It is also possible to obtain plastic and paper holders into which the usual periapical film will slots. Bitewing holders with centring devices are also available. These can be invaluable in any position of the head, but only in mouths where the dentition is even and occlusion normal, as they may not indicate the angulation of the teeth within the arch (Fig. 4.2).

4.4.1 Position of film

In order to prevent extreme discomfort to the patient and consequent lack of co-operation, the upper and lower anterior corners of the bitewing film should be moulded carefully — *not bent* — to the shape of the arches.

The film is then placed downwards into the oral cavity so that the intercrown tab is resting on the crowns of the mandibular teeth. Still with one hand holding the tab to keep good contact between the crowns and film, the patient is advised to close his or her mouth slowly, until the teeth are in occlusion.

In this way, the occlusal plane should be parallel to the horizontal axis of the film and centrally placed. This will demonstrate the maximum number of interproximal spaces.

The inclination of the film towards the mid-line of the hard palate is usually small — about 5–10°. In some instances, such as patients with class III occlusion, it may be as much as 10–15°.

Key points

Bitewings
1. Demonstrate crowns and bone margins
2. Film can be parallel to crowns
3. X-ray beam at 90° to film and crown
4. Film + X-ray beam in used 5–10° to occlusal plane

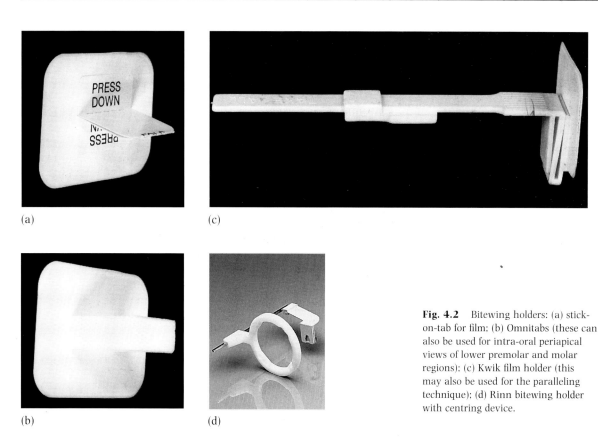

(a)

(c)

(b)

(d)

Fig. 4.2   Bitewing holders: (a) stick-on-tab for film; (b) Omnitabs (these can also be used for intra-oral periapical views of lower premolar and molar regions); (c) Kwik film holder (this may also be used for the paralleling technique); (d) Rinn bitewing holder with centring device.

In other words, when the patient is upright, the downward vertical angulation of the X-ray beam must be adjusted according to the position of the crowns and film. Similarly, it should be adjusted towards the occlusion when horizontal, in the working position (Fig. 4.3).

The horizontal angulation of the X-ray beam is vital to successful bitewing radiography. In order to demonstrate the maximum number of interproximal spaces, the central beam must be directed at right angles to the body of the mandible (Fig. 4.4).

The importance of the horizontal angulation is demonstrated in Fig. 4.5.

The number of films required to show all the interproximal spaces will vary with the regularity of the teeth within the arches. Routinely, one or two films are taken each side to highlight all the spaces between the canine and the third molar. With irregular teeth, however, extra films may be necessary. When the periodontal condition is to be demonstrated, two films should also be taken each side — one film centred for the premolar region, and one for the molar region (Fig. 4.6).

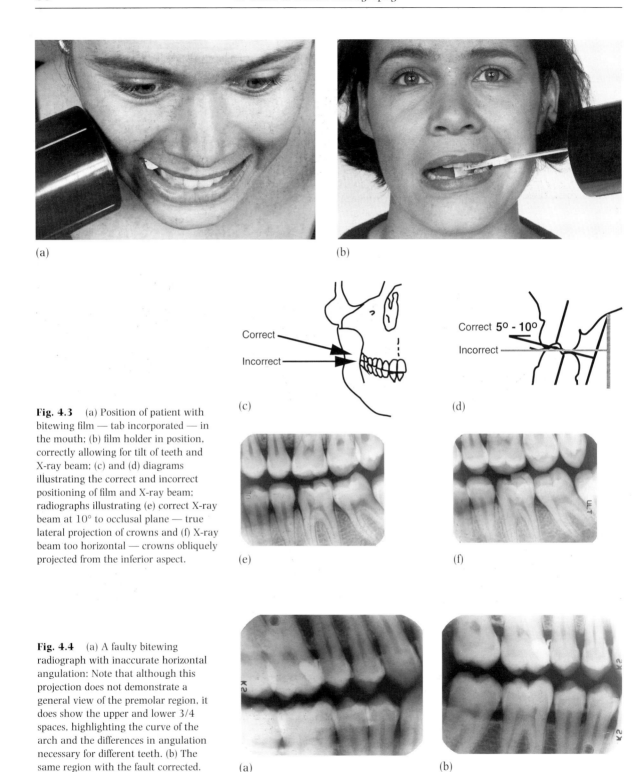

Fig. 4.3 (a) Position of patient with bitewing film — tab incorporated — in the mouth; (b) film holder in position, correctly allowing for tilt of teeth and X-ray beam; (c) and (d) diagrams illustrating the correct and incorrect positioning of film and X-ray beam; radiographs illustrating (e) correct X-ray beam at 10° to occlusal plane — true lateral projection of crowns and (f) X-ray beam too horizontal — crowns obliquely projected from the inferior aspect.

Fig. 4.4 (a) A faulty bitewing radiograph with inaccurate horizontal angulation: Note that although this projection does not demonstrate a general view of the premolar region, it does show the upper and lower 3/4 spaces, highlighting the curve of the arch and the differences in angulation necessary for different teeth. (b) The same region with the fault corrected.

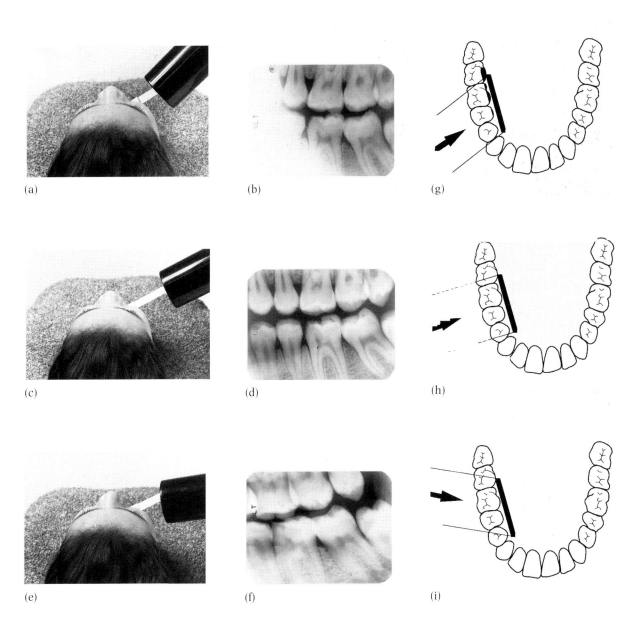

Fig. 4.5 Horizontal alignment of the X-ray beam: (a) too angled from the mesial aspect; (b) X-ray beam centring too far back, with consequent 'cone cutting'; (c) correctly centred; (d) interdental spaces demonstrated; (e) too much angle from the posterior aspect; (f) incorrect angulation causes overlapping of crowns. Diagrams demonstrating the three directional positions of X-ray beam: (g) too far from the mesial aspect; (h) correct; (i) too far from posterior aspect.

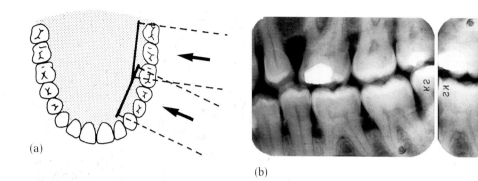

(a)

(b)

Fig. 4.6 Centring points: (a) diagram and (b) two bitewing radiographs taken for periodontal condition of the premolar and molar regions, with different centring points.

4.4.2   Anode–film distance

For all intra-oral radiography, the anode–film distance will depend upon the apparatus but lie somewhere between 20 and 40 cm. Abiding by the Ionising Radiation Regulations, at the present time the radiation field must be limited to 6 cm diameter — but this may be reduced in the future. This limitation emphasizes the advantage of rectangular collimation which considerably reduces the radiation dosage (as recommended in the 1994 Guidelines). Unfortunately, this is not always appropriate or practical.

• It is the responsibility of the general practitioner to limit the field as much possible.

If the anode–film distance is increased, it is very important to increase the exposure factors appropriately (see Chap. 2).

4.4.3   The 3–8 region

When the patient is vertical for bitewing radiography, the position of the head will be as follows:

(1) the sagittal plane is vertical or perpendicular to the floor;

(2) the occlusal plane is horizontal (Fig. 4.7).

When the patient is in the working position, the position of the head will be as follows:

(1) the sagittal plane is central to the longitudinal axis of the chair, and parallel to the floor;

(2) the occlusal plane is vertical (Fig. 4.8a & b).

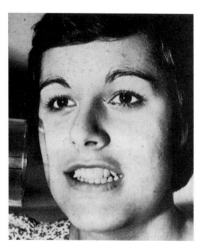

Fig. 4.7   Patient in vertical erect position for bitewing radiograph.

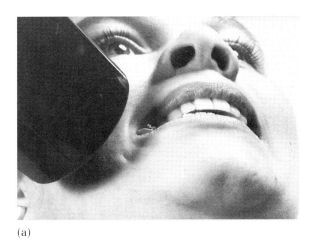
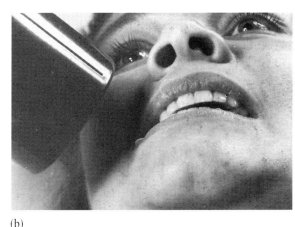

(a)   (b)

Fig. 4.8 (a) Patient in the working position for bitewing radiographs of the molar region — head straight; (b) head rotated towards X-ray tube for the premolar region.

Angulation of the X-ray beam should be 5–10° from the infra-orbital plane, towards the occlusal plane. All centring points should lie along the occlusal plane:

(1) 3–6 regions — 0.5 cm anterior to the line from the outer canthus of the eye, at 90° to the occlusal plane;

(2) 5–8 regions — the point on the occlusal line directly from the outer canthus of the eye.

If a specific interdental space is to be demonstrated, direct the beam through that space. Placement of an interdens massage stick into the interdental space, prior to positioning the X-ray tube, can help to assess how to direct the X-ray beam.

4.4.4 Anterior region

In special instances, to aid diagnosis, it may be necessary to take a bitewing radiograph for anterior teeth, usually for a specific interdental space. It is difficult to place a film near the crowns without excessively bending it.

When the anode–object distance is 20 cm, a small paedodontic film, vertically placed — preferably within a film holder — can be positioned further into the oral cavity. Alternately an extra bitewing tab can be added to the tab already attached. This will increase the object–film distance and so keep the surface of the film at right angles to the X-ray beam and flat. This view can also be taken to demonstrate periodontal disease, where film holders are either not available or unacceptable by the patient (see Fig. 4.14h).

For bitewing radiographs of the anterior region, centre the beam parallel to the space required. When the patient is in a supine position, the important factor is to be sure that the X-ray beam makes the small positive angle downwards, towards the occlusal plane. To demonstrate the interdental spaces, the patient's head may be rotated towards the central beam. This may be easier than moving the tube head laterally (see Fig. 4.8(b)).

4.5   PERIAPICAL, INTRA-ORAL RADIOGRAPHIC TECHNIQUES

Bitewing radiography only produces a lateral projection of the crowns. The next stage is to endeavour to produce a lateral projection of the whole tooth and surrounding bone. In the maxilla, the posterior surface of the alveolar process is continuous with the hard palate. In the lower jaw, the soft tissue formation causes varying depths to the floor of the mouth. These anatomical constraints make it impossible, in almost all cases, to place the film and tooth parallel, and in close proximity. Consequently, there are two techniques for intra-oral radiography of teeth, neither of which is totally satisfactory:

- the parallel film or paralleling technique
- the bisecting angle technique.

The aims of these periapical, intra-oral radiographic techniques are:

(1)   to obtain an image of the whole length of the tooth (from crown to apex of the socket), the surrounding mesial and distal supporting bone structures, and the bone formation beyond the apex;

(2)   to allow for comparative results to aid diagnosis during treatment (for example, endodontics), a period of time (for example, periodontitis), or post-operative bone regeneration;

(3)   to undertake the procedure as swiftly as possible to mimimize the patient's discomfort.

4.6   PARALLELING PERIAPICAL TECHNIQUE

The only way to achieve the ideal situation, with the whole tooth and film parallel, is to place the film further into the oral cavity. To stabilize the film in this position, it is necessary to use film holders. The longest possible anode–object distance should be employed to reduce any consequent magnification (Fig. 4.9). As has been stated, within the radiology departments of dental hospitals, an anode object distance of 40 cm is frequently chosen.

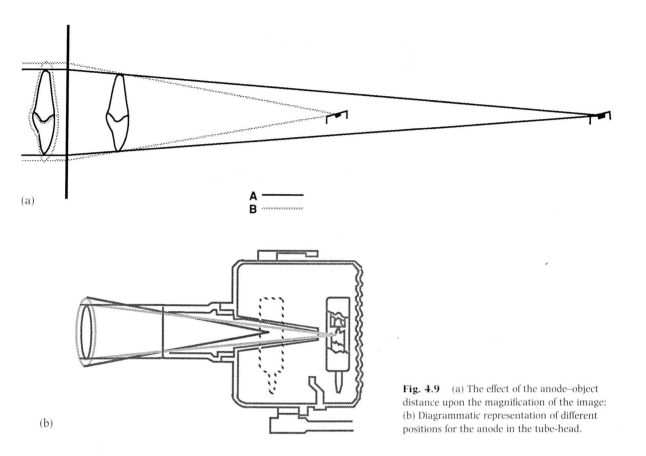

(a)

A ——————
B ···············

(b)

Fig. 4.9 (a) The effect of the anode–object distance upon the magnification of the image; (b) Diagrammatic representation of different positions for the anode in the tube-head.

In general dental practice, the colloquially named 'long cone' (the expression 'long cone' is now an anachronism) gives an anode-object distance often of only 20 cm. This is still twice the length of the old, low kilovoltage (50–60 kV) apparatus, when the anode object distance was only 10 cms. 'Cone' goes back historically to old apparatus with plastic centering devices, now no longer acceptable under IRR 1985.

There is dental apparatus which allows a 35–40 cm anode–film distance with a conventional length collimating device. It achieves this by placing the X-ray tube at the far end of the tube head.

The Heliodent MD also has the X-ray tube at the far end of the tube head, making a very compact tube head — but the anode-film distance is only 20 cm (Fig. 4.10). Practically, diagnostic results, with good detail, are achievable with the 20 cm anode–object distance.

The relationship between the object and the film controls the magnification factor: it is a geometric problem, and the magnification can be decreased by using smaller films in some areas to reduce the object–film distance, for example, for anterior teeth. In this case, the narrowness of the arches means that standard dental film would have to go even further into the mouth (Fig. 4.11).

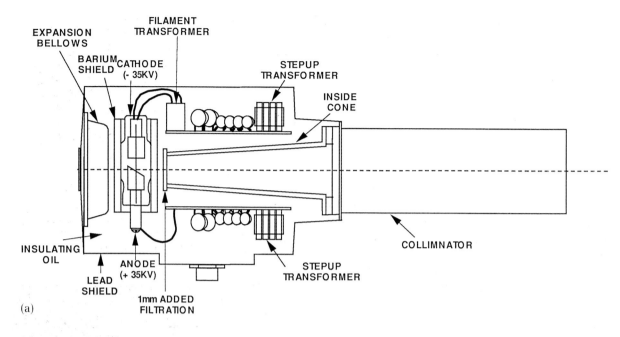

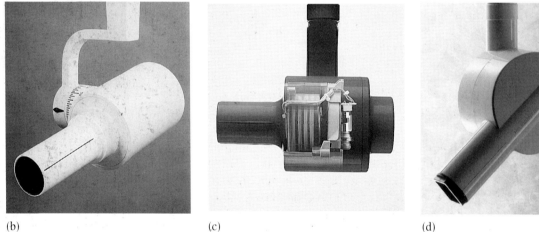

(b)   (c)   (d)

Fig. 4.10   (a) Diagrammatic position of the anode at the rear of the X-ray tube behind the transformer in the modern Keystone dental X-ray apparatus; (b) Schick Keystone Discovery tube head; (c) Heliodent MD tube head showing position of the X-ray tube; (d) Heliodent tube head with rectangular collimation.

Paralleling periapical technique has differing degrees of success in different dental regions:

1.   It is most difficult to achieve success in the upper canine and the first premolar regions.

2. It works well for the upper molars, where it prevents the superimposition of the zygoma.

3. In the lower molar region, where the tooth and film are parallel, there is no problem.

4.6.1 Requirements: of X-ray apparatus and collimating devices

For the film and object to be parallel, it is necessary to place the film further into the mouth, and so increase the object–film distance. It is, therefore, impractical to attempt this technique with apparatus which does not have at least a 20 cm anode–film distance, that is, apparatus operating above 60 kVp (usually 65–75 kVp fixed output). If the apparatus offers an option of a longer 30–40 cm anode distance, remember to increase the exposure factors.

As it is necessary to use film holders, in order to maintain the position of the film within the mouth as parallel to the teeth, it is usual to add a centring device to the film holder. This should be positioned in a constant relationship to the skin, to standardize the exposure factors. To comply with the Code of Practice, the anode–object distance should not be increased so much that the field of irradiation at the skin surface is greater than 6 cm diameter.

4.6.2 Mechanical film holders with collimating devices (Fig. 4.12)

1. Precision film holders limit the field of irradiation at the same time as increasing the anode distance. They are ideal for use with the 20 cm collimating device. These metal holders give rectangular film collimation and increase the effective anode-film distance to 30 cm. They have their own plastic disposable biting pads, and may have an advantage in that the patient can help maintain the position of the holder manually. It is not necessary to rely only upon occlusion. There is a set of three holder — for all of the month — four, if the paedodontic size film is incorporated.

2. Rinn parallel film holders, with their centring aids, had plastic, and now have disposable polystyrene biting blocks — the cost of which may be a contra-indication. The centring devices need to be accurately aligned.

Both these film holders, and the metal precision holders, incorporate means for aligning the collimating devices and the tube head.

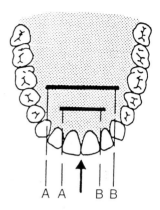

Fig. 4.11 The object–film distance: (a) standard size periapical film; (b) paedodontic size periapical film.

Key points

Paralleling intra-oral technique
1. Tooth and film should be parallel
2. X-ray beam at 90° to tooth and film
3. Anode–film distance, preferably 40 cm, but 20 cm acceptable
4. Accurate collimation essential — diameter of field of irradiation, 6 cm maximum
5. Film holders, necessary
6. Collimating devices, helpful

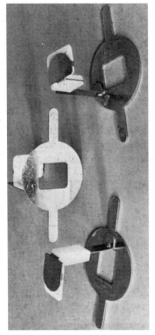
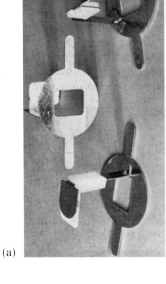

(a)

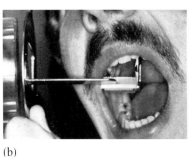

(b)

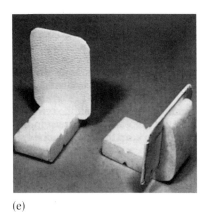

(e)

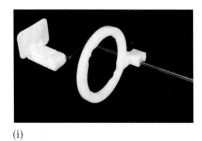

(i)

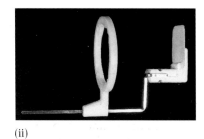

(ii)

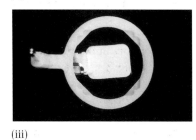

(iii)

(c)

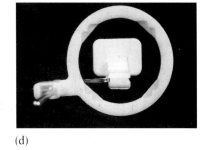

(d)

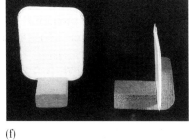

(f)

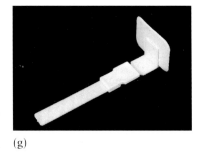

(g)

Fig. 4.12 Film holders: (a) Precision metal film holders designed to give rectangular film collimation; (b) Metal holder positioned in the mouth for the upper premolars; (c) Rinn film holders with centring devices; (d) Rinn film holders with centring aids; (e) Stable disposable polystyrene film holders for the paralleling or long-anode technique — can also be used for the bisecting angle technique with the end removed; (f) Simple wooden film holders; (g) Kwik holder, with film placed for the paralleling technique.

3. Film holders without an extra centring device for aligning the X-ray beam include:

— disposable polystyrene holders
— wooden bite block holders
— plastic film holders

4. Special rectangular collimating systems are also available for a minimum field of irradiation.

These types of film holder are recommended in the 1994 Guidelines (NRPB 1994). Although use of the rectangular collimator is to be encouraged, there are instances where is not appropriate.

For use with the Rinn film holders, an adapter can now be added to the end of the round X-ray tube collimator, to reduce the field to the rectangular field and thus cut down on the irradiation (Fig. 4.13).

• It is very important with this rectangular collimator to be sure that the aperture is correctly rotated so that the long axis is horizontally or vertically in line with the film.

A film holder should be chosen for the comfort and accuracy of its placement in the mouth, and how speedily the X-ray beam can be centred. Some operators prefer the simple holder, and rely on the accuracy of their eye to align the X-ray beam and the collimator. This is usually the quickest method, but it needs expertise and, whilst it is acceptable with an 20 cm anode distance, it is almost impossible with 40 cm.

Other operators prefer film-holders with built-in centring devices. These tend to lengthen the procedure, but assist in the centring of the X-ray beam. In order to keep the film flat, all these film holders give solid support behind most of the film area. Unfortunately, this is uncomfortable for the patient. In order to achieve maximum co-operation, it is worth spending time explaining why this technique is considered valuable for both the dentist and, consequently, the patient. When placing the film holder into the mouth, ease the patient gently from the horizontal to the lateral position.

As there is minimal enlargement, it is possible, in most cases, to raise the crowns off the edge of the film holder with a cotton wool roll and still project the apex on to the film (Fig. 4.14c).

Great care must be taken in the correct positioning of the film to ensure that it is parallel to the long axis of the tooth. The mouth should be examined carefully to judge exactly where to place the film. If the film is not placed sufficiently far into the oral cavity, then the apices of the teeth may not be included on the film.

Sometimes, true parallelism is impossible to achieve due to anatomical difficulties (see Fig. 4.14b). When this is the case for the whole

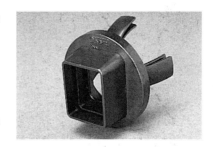

Fig. 4.13   Adapter for restricting round collimator to rectangular — designed to be used with Rinn round collimating devices.

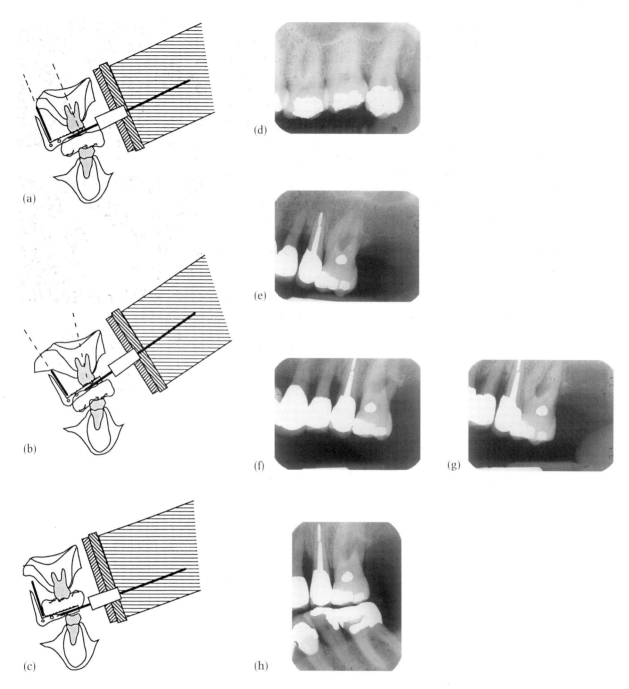

Fig. 4.14 Paralleling intra-oral technique. Diagrams showing: (a) correct position of tooth and film; (b) film and tooth not parallel, due to a low arch producing foreshortened image; (c) raised crown, with a cotton wool roll to lift tooth off the holder — allows true paralleling for periodontal assessment. Radiographs showing: (d) high vault allowing for true paralleling; (e) low arch not allowing true paralleling — foreshortening of tooth; (f) raised crown demonstrating pocketing round 1st premolar; (g) lateral angulation changed — this time demonstrating infra bony pocket; (h) vertical bitewing, for same problem.

tooth, and only the periodontal condition is required, then a compromise is necessary by placing a cotton wool roll below the crowns and accepting the fact that the apex will not be demonstrated (see Fig. 4.14c). If the whole tooth is to be demonstrated, then another technique must be used (see Ch. 16).

The X-ray beam must always be at right angles to the film. The easiest way to assess if this is so is to place the plane of the collimator at the skin surface, parallel to the film, if centring devices are not incorporated. If they are, then special care must be taken to ensure that the end of the device is really accurately aligned (Fig. 4.15). The angulation in the horizontal plane is of vital importance in order to prevent overlapping of teeth, the obscuring of the interproximal spaces, and lack of information as to the periodontal condition. These principles are the same as for bitewing radiography.

Sometimes, the film and holder are parallel with the tooth, not the bony contour of the arch.

The margin of error is small and, for example, the upper canine and incisor region tends to necessitate the taking of more films with this technique, than with the bisecting technique (see Fig. 4.23).

Where the arch is very narrow, the small 2.2 × 3.5 cm film, vertically placed, may be easier to position into the mouth. The larger film will inevitably lead to some distortion due to bending of the film to fit the patient's arch and for greater comfort. This may also apply in the mandible.

Position of head

The sagittal plane should always be carefully assessed, whether in the vertical or the supine position. In the horizontal position, the central beam will always be at right angles to the film anyway. The head should be comfortably immobilized.

Centring points

With careful placement of the film, the central beam can be directed to the centre of the tooth or teeth under examination, at a point level with the gum margin. (Obviously, a judgement has to be made when gum margins recede.)

4.6.3 Placement of film

Mandibular regions

In all the mandibular regions, the film and film holder should be slowly and gently eased into place and the patient reassured that as he or she closes on to the bite block, the floor of the mouth will relax. Where the mouth is narrow, the use of 2.2 × 3.5 cm film, carefully

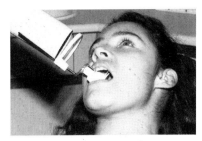

(a)

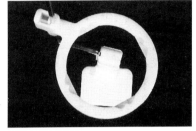

(b)

Fig. 4.15   (a) Incorrect alignment of the centring device; (b) effect of this error on the collimator–film relationship. Differing interdental relationships can cause errors in diagnosis.

placed vertically in the film holder will allow parallelism to be achieved more easily in the more anterior teeth, but it does necessitate *perfect placement* of the film.

Lower molars

The film should be placed with its long axis into the film holder, so that the biting block is to the anterior corner of the film, if possible. The film may be placed in contact with the mandible behind the molar region — so paralleling should not be a problem (Fig. 4.16).

Lower premolars

The film should be placed with its long axis into the film holder, the biting block in the centre; the film must be placed under the tongue, with a small gap between the film and the premolars which are positioned towards the centre of the film.

Sometimes, it is easier to place the film vertically and use a cotton wool roll below the holder. The anterior corner can be moulded to prevent discomfort (Fig. 4.17).

Lower canines

The film should be placed with its short axis into the film holder. Use a cotton wool roll between the biting block and the crowns of the teeth to ease the placement of the film into the floor of the mouth.

This is an area where parallelism is difficult to obtain; a slight angle between the teeth and film may be necessary. There will be a gap between the canine, which is centrally positioned, and the film (Fig. 4.18).

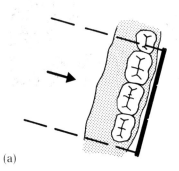
(a)

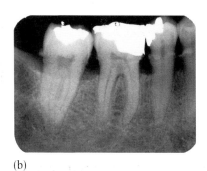
(b)

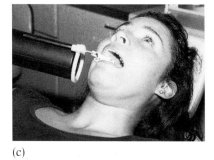
(c)

Fig. 4.16 Parallel film periapical technique for lower molars: (a) position of the film for the lower molar teeth, from the occlusal aspect; (b) radiograph; (c) patient in the working position.

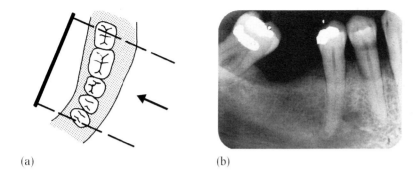

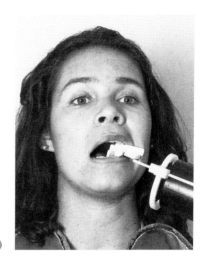

Fig. 4.17 Parallel film periapical technique for lower premolars:
(a) position of the film for the lower premolar teeth, from the occlusal aspect;
(b) radiograph; (c) patient in the vertical position.

(c)

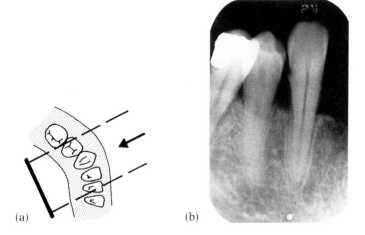

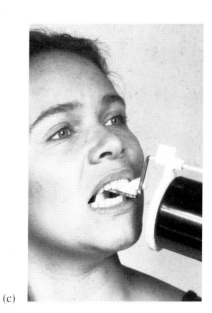

Fig. 4.18 Parallel film periapical technique for lower canines: (a) position of
the film for the lower canine teeth, from the occlusal aspect; (b) radiograph;
(c) patient in the vertical position.

(c)

Lower incisors

The film is placed with its short axis into the film holder. Use a cotton
wool roll, as with the canines, to ease the placement of the film which
needs to be positioned as far back as possible under the tongue
(Fig. 4.19).

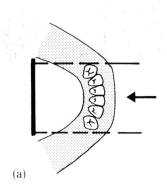

(a)

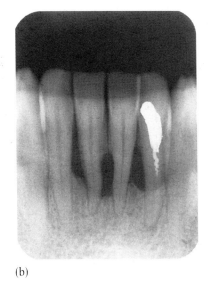

(b)

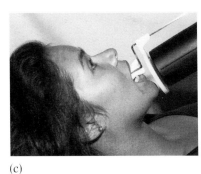

(c)

Fig. 4.19   Parallel film periapical technique for lower incisors: (a) position of the film for the lower incisor teeth, from the occlusal aspect; (b) radiograph; (c) patient in the working position; (d) patient in the vertical position.

(d)

Maxillary regions

In all maxillary regions, if the patient is required to bite to retain the film in a position, a cotton wool roll below the film holder and the mandibular teeth makes the occlusion more stable.

Upper molars

The film is placed with the long axis into the film holder, so that the biting block is to the anterior corner of the film, if possible. This is the most comfortable position of the film for the patient but can present problems, for example, with the rectangular collimation centring device.

- It is important to place the film so that it is square to the inter-dental spaces, if the periodontal condition is to be diagnosed.
- This position may not always coincide with the contour of the maxilla. The direction of the X-ray beam must be adjusted accordingly. As with bitewing radiography, individual spaces may need individual radiographs (Fig. 4.20).

Upper premolars

The film is placed with the long axis into the film holder, and beyond the lateral axes of the premolars. The teeth are placed as centrally as possible on the film. As with the lower premolars, a small film placed, vertically, more to the midline of the palate, may be more acceptable to the patient.

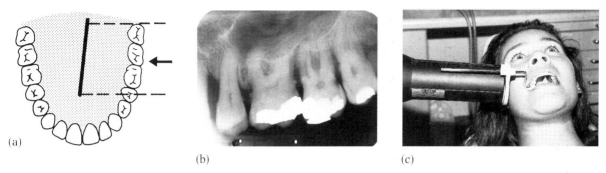

(a) (b) (c)

Fig. 4.20 Parallel film periapical technique for upper molars: (a) position of the film for the upper molar teeth, from the occlusal aspect; (b) radiograph; (c) patient in the working position.

- Care must be taken, however to ensure that the film is parallel to both the long and lateral axes of these teeth (Fig. 4.21).

Upper canines
The film is placed with its short side into the film holder and positioned centrally, behind the canine, but far into the oral cavity. *The apex of this tooth may incline towards the first premolar* (Fig. 4.22).

Upper incisors
Usually, three films are taken in this region — two lateral centrals, and one midline. In some arches, a separate film may by needed for each incisor. The film is placed with its short side into the film holder, behind each tooth to be examined, well into the mouth. In the midline position, it is approximately level with the first molar (Fig. 4.23).

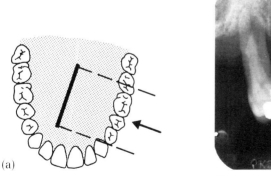
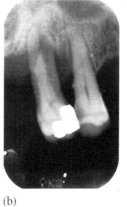
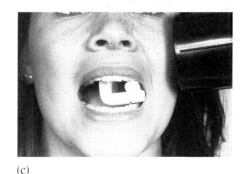

(a) (b) (c)

Fig. 4.21 Parallel film periapical technique for upper premolars: (a) position of the film for the upper premolar teeth, from the occlusal aspect; (b) radiograph; (c) patient in the vertical position using a Stabe film holder.

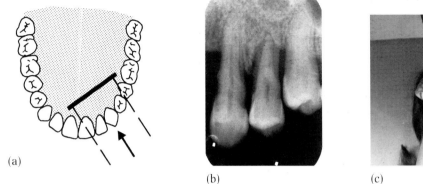

Fig. 4.22   Parallel film periapical technique for upper canines: (a) position of the film for the upper canine teeth, from the occlusal aspect; (b) radiograph; (c) patient in the working position: note the rotation of the head towards the tube.

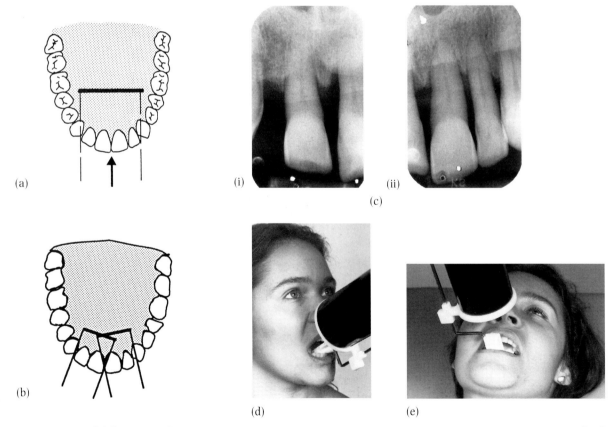

Fig. 4.23   Parallel film periapical technique for upper incisors: (a) position of the film for the upper incisor teeth, from the occlusal aspect; (b) position of two narrow films, shortening the object-film distance; (c) radiographs demonstrating the incisors on two films; (d) patient in the vertical position, and (e) patient in the working position.

4.6.4 General considerations

Unfortunately, there are some patients who are unsuitable for the paralleling intra-oral technique due to anatomical contraints or their inability to co-operate adequately. *This may occur when the patient is in pain because of trauma or infection.* It may also occur when the patient is apprehensive or communication is difficult. In these cases, the other standard intra-oral technique may be more appropriate.

REFERENCES AND FURTHER READING

Brocklebank, L. (1997). *Dental radiology — understanding the X-ray image.* Oxford University Press, Oxford.

Waite, E. (1996). *Essentials of dental radiography and radiology* (2nd edn). Churchill Livingstone.

Haring, J.I. (1996). *Dental radiography: principles and techniques.* W.B. Saunders.

Frommer, H.H. (1987). *Radiology for dental auxiliaries* (4th edn). C.V. Mosby, St Louis.

Goaz, P.W. and White, S.C. (1987). *Oral radiology — principles and interpretation* (2nd edn). C.V. Mosby, St Louis.

Manon-Hing, L.R. (1985). *Fundamentals of dental radiography* (2nd edn) Lea and Febiger, Philadelphia.

Perlman, C. (1973). *A student guide for dental radiography.* The University of Texas Dental Branch, Houston.

Updegrave, W.J. (1971). *New horizons in periapical and interproximal radiography.* Rinn Corporation, Illinois.

Rinn Corporation (1989). *Intra-oral radiography with Rinn XCP/BIA Instruments.* Rinn Corporation, Illinois.

Weissman, D.D. (1973). *Manual of rectangular field collimation for intra-oral periapical radiography.* The University of California, Los Angeles.

NRPB. (1994). *Guidelines on radiology standards for primary dental care.*

5 Intra-oral radiography: II

5.1 BISECTING ANGLE TECHNIQUE

5.1.1 Introduction

This easily achievable and adaptable technique is the one that has been most commonly used in dental practice since the beginnings of dental radiography. It was an essential technique to use with 'low output' dental X-ray apparatus with an anode–object distance of 10 cm, but even better results are obtained with longer anode–object distances, as there is less enlargement. (See Ch. 4 for details of anode–object distances.)

The intra-oral film is placed behind the palatal or lingual aspects of the teeth in apposition. Close contact between the whole tooth and the film cannot be promoted, as the root (two-thirds) of the tooth is embedded in the alveolar process and, in most instances, this will produce an angle between the film and the tooth, and subsequent image projection problems:

1. If the central ray of the X-ray beam is directed at right angles to the long axis of the tooth, the image is elongated (Fig. 5.1).
2. If the central ray of the X-ray beam is directed ar right angles to the long axis of the film, the image is foreshortened (Fig. 5.2).
3. A compromise is reached by directing the central beam at right angles to an imaginary plane bisecting the angle made by the film and tooth (Fig. 5.3).

The variations in the anatomical contours of both upper and lower arches, combined with the differing inclination of the teeth within them, will give a wide range of angles between the tooth and film. This makes comparative work difficult and also slows down the procedure if each film needs individual assessment.

To combat these problems and to isolate the patient's individual anatomical variations, it is recommended that as many factors as possible are standardized.

One is then able to describe this technique in a formal way, which is both easy to learn and perform.

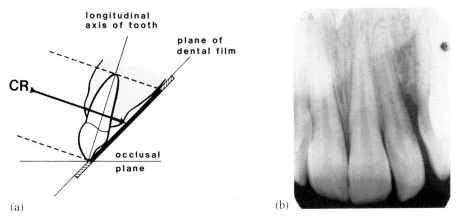

Fig. 5.1 When the central ray is projected at right angles to the long axis of the tooth (a) the image is elongated (b).

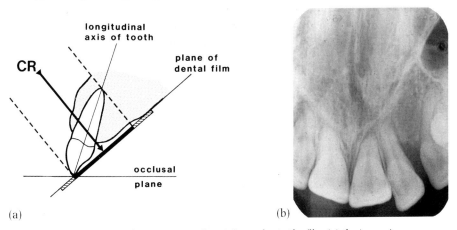

Fig. 5.2 When the central ray is projected at right angles to the film (a) the image is shortened (b).

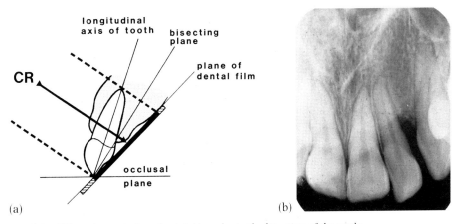

Fig. 5.3 When the central ray is at right angles to the bisection of the angle between the object and the film (a) the image results with the minimum distortion (b).

Usually, bisecting angle technique is initially undertaken in the dental imaging department, or with X-ray apparatus in a radiation protected room within a dental school, with the dental chair in the upright position. Adaptation of this technique to the working position will be after the basic principles have been understood. These include the fact that

- The position of the head, which effectively means the position of the tooth, must remain constant. It is then possible to plot the centring points on one line.
- Familiarity with the positions of the head will make angulation and directions of the X-ray beam easier to assess. Combining this assessment with facial skin marking makes it easy to centre the X-ray beam from the external aspect (Fig. 5.4).

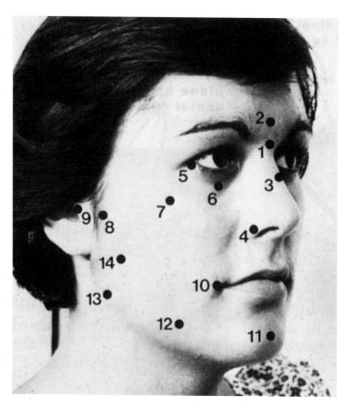

Fig. 5.4 Skin surface landmarks useful in intra-oral radiography: (1) nasion; (2) glabella; (3) bridge of nose; (4) ala of nose; (5) outer canthus of eye; (6) midpoint of infra-orbital margin; (7) zygomatic bone; (8) temporomandibular articulation; (9) tragus of ear; (10) corner of mouth; (11) symphysis menti; (12) body of mandible; (13) angle of mandible; (14) ramus of mandible.

• This is especially useful in the molar regions, when having to look inside the mouth again, to centre the beam after placement of the film, slows down the procedure.

5.1.2 Positioning of the head with the patient erect

The teeth and alveolar processes are units of the facial bones, which are themselves fixed components of the skull. If the head is stabilized, the position of the teeth is automatically standardized. Required positions are:

(1) vertical plane: position the head, with the help of the head support, so that the sagittal plane is vertical and at right angles to the floor;

(2) horizontal or occlusal plane:

  (a) maxilla — lower the patient's chin so that an imaginary line, drawn from the ala of the nose to the tragus of the ear, is parallel to the floor (Fig. 5.5(a)). The back of the chair or head support should be raised, to push the occipital region of the head forwards, to maintain this position. Insert foam pads if necessary between the head and chair cushions;

  (b) mandible — lower the chair back and raise the patient's chin so that an imaginary line, drawn from the angle of the mouth to the tragus of the ear, is parallel to the floor (Fig. 5.5(b).

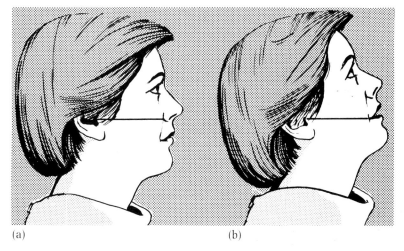

(a)   (b)

Fig. 5.5 Correct position of the head for (a) the maxillary teeth and (b) the mandibular teeth.

This is useful as a guide-line but it is the occlusal surfaces of the teeth that must be horizontal in the erect position, and the exact position of these will be particular to each patient. The occlusal surfaces of the teeth will be the constants when the head is in the working position and the occlusal plane is vertical.

The position of the head using the the occlusal surfaces of the teeth as the horizontal plane, combined with extra-oral (skin surface) landmarks, has two important advantages:

(1)   there is a baseline to measure and control vertical angulation;

(2)   it aids the centring of the X-ray beam as it orientates the tooth in the vertical position, highlighting the apex.

This is important, as many errors occur in horizontal angulation. Once the film is correctly placed behind the teeth, it should not be necessary to look inside the mouth again.

Because of the horseshoe shape of the dental arches, it is seldom possible to get more than two teeth in the same plane. Therefore, it is necessary to divide each quadrant into four regions: incisor, canine, premolar, and molar.

When inserting the film into the mouth, the margin carrying the small embossment (marked on the outside of the dental film packet) should be placed towards the crowns. Though this procedure is not essential to good radiography, it is a useful habit to acquire, for it will assist staff to identify and mount the films after processing.

In accordance with the recommendations of the Code of Practice for the Protection of Persons against Ionizing Radiation arising from any Work Activity (1985), the use of open-ended cylindrical or retangular (1994 Guidelines) collimators are necessary and *must be* encouraged.

Apart from the obvious protection advantage, use of such collimators makes it necessary for the operator to check the centring points from two aspects — vertical and horizontal. This is essential for correct alignment of the X-ray beam.

If placed just off the skin surface, the collimating applicator will also maintain a constant anode–film distance and outline the diameter of the beam on the skin.

5.1.3 Film holders

The use of film holders is strongly recommended — though not essential — in the bisecting angle technique:

1.   It will eliminate any irradiation to the patient's hand.

2.   It will keep the object–film relationship constant for any particular tooth. This is of enormous value when comparable radiographs are required.

3. The most common fault in dental radiography is distortion due to curvature of the film, mainly caused by the pressure of the patient's finger or thumb.

4. It is often difficult to maintain the position of the film in the mouth without this pressure, particularly in the maxilla. Film holders will help to keep the film flat and in position but, even so, they must be used carefully. (See Figs 5.7(b)).

5. When it is difficult to obtain patient co-operation, either because of extreme age or nerves, film holders make the effort of maintaining the film in the correct position, intra-orally, far simpler. This is especially so in the mandible, where the floor of the mouth relaxes as it closes, and the lower border of the film does not cause so much discomfort. In any case, to tell a patient to bite down on to a holder, despite discomfort, seems to elicit more co-operation than to ask him or her to hold a film down into the floor of the mouth with a finger. So often, the film rises high above the crowns before the exposure is made, and the apex may not be demonstrated (see Ch. 16).

6. The positive action of biting on to to a film holder also helps the patient to conquer the impulse to gag. This can occur, in some patients, in almost any dental region but, in most patients, chiefly with the third molars.

7. Film holders will help the patient to keep still during centring of the X-ray beam and consequent exposure of the film — to be immobile, with one arm in the air holding a film into the mouth, is difficult.

The simplest film holder consists of a wood, polystyrene, or plastic biting block, with a groove and support for the film. The film is inserted into the groove and the patient bites upon the biting block. In order not to traumatize the incisor edges of the crowns of the teeth, cotton wool rolls may be interposed on one or both sides of the biting block. This also provides a firmer bite and raises the incisive margins of the teeth from the edge of the film. This is particularly important when the X-ray beam angulation is high, as with central incisors, when the crowns could be projected off the film. The film can be placed into the film holder in the vertical or horizontal axis — as appropriate to the tooth under examination and the shape of the dental arch (Figs 5.6 and 5.7).

5.1.4 Placement of the film into the mouth

To ensure that the image of the entire tooth appears on the radiograph, care must be taken when positioning the film. If it is introduced

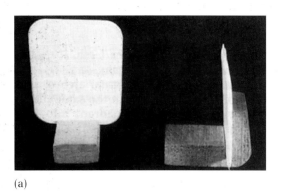 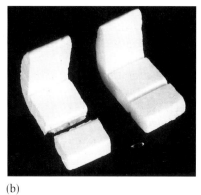

(a)   (b)

Fig. 5.6   (a) Simple film holders made of wood (Mason film holders). The long or short side of the film may be placed into the holder which gives support on the non-tube side. There are three surfaces upon which the patient may bite, depending on the angulation of the film to the tooth. There are three sizes available; (b) Stabe holder, shortened for the bisecting angle technique.

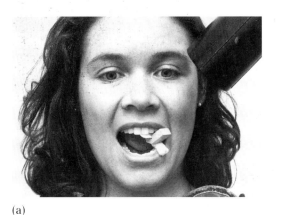 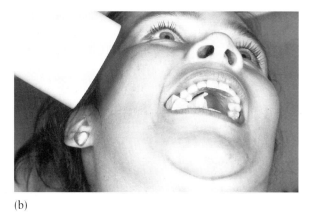

(a)   (b)

Fig. 5.7   (a) Film holder in the mouth, for the upper canine region; (b) film holder in the mouth, demonstrating that, even with film holders, care must be taken not to bend the film.

into the mouth in the occlusal plane, and the crown is correctly placed, then the film may be gently angled towards the apex. Position of the crown should be as follows:

(1) for the incisors, it is parallel with the short edge of the film;

(2) for the molars, it is parallel with the long edge of the film;

(3) in the canine region, it should lie upon the diagonal;

(4) in the premolar region, it should lie diagonally or horizontally, as appropriate.

Never allow the film to be so close to the arch that it curves into its contour. Also, Always keep the film flat behind the tooth to be examined, even when it is necessary to mould the anterior corner of the film so it is as high or as low in the arch as possible, for example, for premolars and the first molar teeth. Ease of positioning, not the length of the tooth, should govern the way the film goes into the mouth. Seldom will the image of a tooth be even 3 cm long, that is, as long as the short side of the film.

If film holders cannot be used, for example, during endodontic treatment, then place the patient's forefinger, from the opposite side, against the crown. There are now some holders on the market, made especially to accommodate the endodontic situation (see Fig 6.9).

- Do not hesitate to incorporate cotton wool rolls between the tooth and film, to help keep the film flat when film holders are not used. They lessen the curvature of the film which occurs with the pressure of the patient's finger (see Fig. 5.18(c)).

5.1.4 Angulation and direction of the X-ray beam

The X-ray beam should be centred to the midpoint of the tooth to be examined. All centring points will lie on the same plane, known as the 'line of concentration' which:

(1) for maxillary teeth can be judged to be the ala-tragal line;

(2) for mandibular teeth can be judged to be 1 cm above the border of the mandible.

The central ray of the X-ray beam is directed at right angles to the bisection of the tooth and film. In the lower third molar, the film and tooth are usually parallel, and so the X-ray beam can be horizontal. The angle between the teeth and film rises gradually coming round the incisor region, when the angle of the central beam will increase to $-25°$. In the maxilla, the central ray should be about $+20°$ in the molar region, again increasing — due to the enlarging angle between the teeth and film — round the incisor region, to about $55°$.

The angle between the teeth and film will depend upon the height of the dome of the palate and the depth of the floor of the mouth. The higher the dome, the smaller the angle between tooth and film and, therefore, the lower the angle of the central beam (Fig. 5.8).

The angle of incidence is increased both early and late in life — in the absence of the alveolar process, either through non-development or non-eruption of the teeth in children, or in the edentulous patient with resorption of the process.

In these circumstances, the film would tend to lie more horizontally in relation to the occlusal planes and, with retained roots, would need

Key points

Bisecting angle technique
- film in contact with crown and palatal or lingual aspect of dental arch
- Xray-beam bisects angle between tooth and film

Standard position of head
- ala-tragal or occlusal plane 90° to sagittal plane advantages
- position of teeth remain constant
- able to localise centering points
- able to centre X-ray beam without looking in mouth
- and check alignment from vertical and horizontal aspects
- base line to measure and control angulation

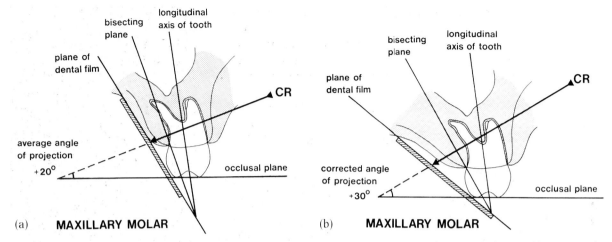

Fig. 5.8 (a) A high vault requires approximately +20°angulation in the upper molar region; (b) a low vault requires approximately +30° angulation in the upper molar region.

special consideration. If only deciduous teeth are to be examined, then small films may be used which will allow teeth and film to be more nearly parallel. In these cases, the angle of incidence can be decreased 5–10° from the average adult angle.

Edentulous areas

When retained roots are to be demonstrated in edentulous patients, it is helpful to place a cotton wool roll between the alveolar process and the film, as well as between the ridge and film holder. This will allow the film and the object to make a smaller angle, and so a lower angle of incidence may be used, thus demonstrating the alveolar ridge without superimposition of inferior and superior bone. There will be a slight increase of the object–film distance but this is usually compensated for by a decrease in the angle between the film and alveolar process. Exposure factors, too, will need reducing.

Another method for edentulous areas in the lower premolar and molar regions involves an adaptation of the bitewing film, filling the upper space with a cotton wool roll. In the mandible, a small film may again be more comfortable.

Tooth inclination:

(1) the proclined tooth will need a greater degree of angulation than normal;

(2) the retroclined tooth will need less angulation of the central beam (see Ch. 6 for anatomical variations.)

It is very important that the X-ray beam comes in horizontally, at right angles to the tangent at the area of the jaw under examination, regardless of the rotation of the tooth within the alveolar process.

This will minimize the widening or narrowing of the tooth shadow and prevent overlapping of the shadows of the crowns and roots of adjoining teeth (Fig. 5.9).

This principle always applies for intra-oral radiography, (see the illustrations for bitewing radiography—Fig. 4.5), although an adaptation of the angulation is utilized to separate multi-rooted teeth (Fig. 5.19).

Key points

Filmholders
- eliminate radiation to hand
- keep object–film relationship constant
- eliminate or control curvature of film
- helps patient co-operation

Placement of film in mouth
- case film and holder behind crown towards apex
- to keep film flat — corner may be moulded
- incorporate cotton-wool rolls if no film holder available

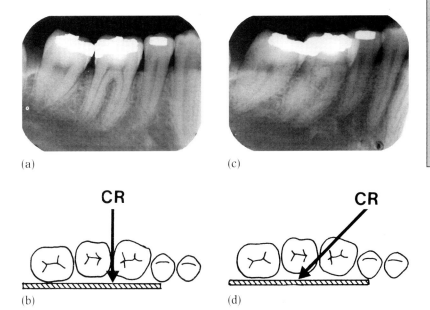

(a)

(c)

(b)

(d)

Fig. 5.9 (a) (b) When the central beam is projected at the correct horizontal angle, the images are distinct, and overlapping is avoided; (c) (d) when the central ray is projected at an incorrect horizontal angle, the images are badly overlapping and blurred.

5.1.5 Application of technique to specific regions

Lower molar region

It is seldom possible to get the three molar teeth on one film, as the roots of the third molar tend to incline distally — a second film may need to be taken. Place the film with the long axis horizontally in the mouth, behind the molar teeth, so that the upper edge is 2 mm above the crowns.

- *Centring point*: 3 cm anterior to the angle of the mandible; cm above the lower border.

- *Angulation*: 0 to –10°.
- *Anode–film distance*: 20 cm
(Fig. 5.10 (a) and (b))

Lower molars can have additional roots and root canals. For endodontic purposes, this necessitates careful assessment of the beam direction, with variations in the horizontal or lateral angulation to separate and so demonstrate these roots (see Fig. 5.10(c) and (d)).

Under these conditions, the lack of clarity of the periapical tissues is not important, provided that the contrast is sufficient to identify the root apex from the surrounding bone (Fig. 6.9(e), Ch. 6).

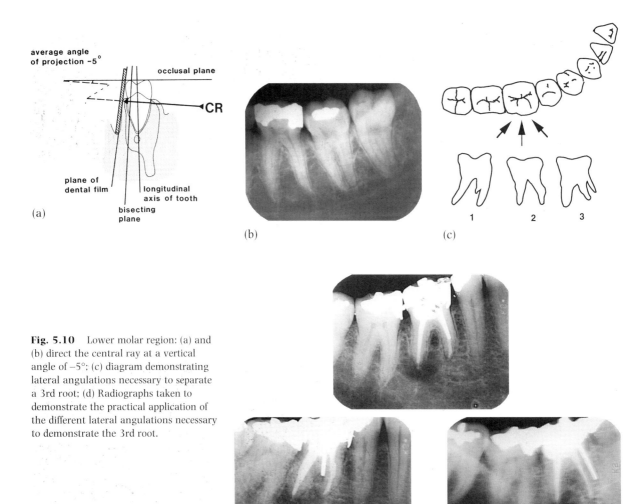

Fig. 5.10   Lower molar region: (a) and (b) direct the central ray at a vertical angle of –5°; (c) diagram demonstrating lateral angulations necessary to separate a 3rd root; (d) Radiographs taken to demonstrate the practical application of the different lateral angulations necessary to demonstrate the 3rd root.

Unerupted third molar

The Worth or Alan film holder is especially useful in this area. Place the clip slightly diagonally at the upper anterior corner of the film, in case of an impacting tooth. Lower the film and holder gently down the side of the tongue — so that the anterior corner of the film is about half-way along the crown of the first molar.

Speed is essential in centring the X-ray beam, as the patient will find this a difficult film to retain in the mouth; and gagging is a problem.

When correctly positioned and retained by the film holder, the floor of the mouth becomes relaxed giving the patient minimum discomfort (Figs 5.11 and 5.12).

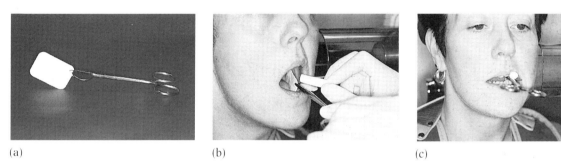

(a)   (b)   (c)

Fig. 5.11   Technique for third molars: (a) Spencer-Wells, with metal semi-circular horizontal projection added, placed diagonally on the corner of the film; (b) film placed into the mouth with cotton wool roll to ensure firm occlusion; (c) patient in vertical position with holder and film in place.

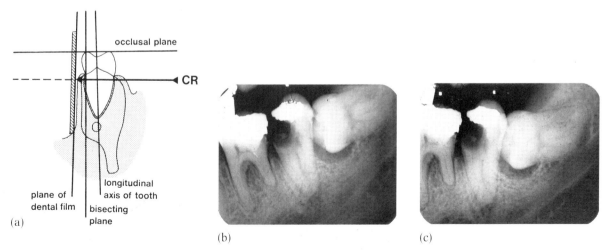

(a)   (b)   (c)

Fig. 5.12   (a) Lower 3rd molar region, beam directed horizontally; (b) film with long axis horizontal; (c) long axis diagonal, for impacted third molar.

- *Centring point*: 2 cm anterior to the angle of the mandible; 1 cm above the lower border
- *Angulation*: 0°
- *Anode–film distance*: 20 cm

Lower premolar region

Place the film, with the long axis horizontally, in the mouth so that 2 mm of it is above the crowns and the premolars are in the centre. This will necessitate moulding the lower anterior corner of the film to the curvature of the mandible. Never try to place the film vertically down into the floor of the mouth, as this causes discomfort to the patient but, in some narrow arches, the film may be placed diagonally. In these cases, the angle between the tooth and the film will be increased with the consequent increase of the X-ray beam angulation.

Always place the film obliquely under the tongue and gradually bring into contact with the lingual aspects of the teeth.

- *Centring point*: line down from the angle of the mouth, when open, 1 cm above the lower border
- *Angulation*: –10 to –15°
- *Anode-film distance*: 20 cm

(Fig. 5.13)

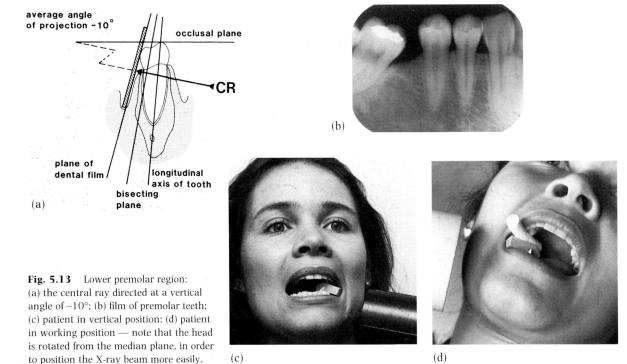

Fig. 5.13 Lower premolar region: (a) the central ray directed at a vertical angle of –10°; (b) film of premolar teeth; (c) patient in vertical position; (d) patient in working position — note that the head is rotated from the median plane, in order to position the X-ray beam more easily.

Lower canine region

The film is placed in the mouth diagonally, behind the long axis of the tooth, with the upper edge 5 mm above the crown. Care must be taken to avoid excessive curvature of the film.

- It is always better to make a bigger angle between the tooth and the film, and keep the film flat (Ch. 6, Fig. 6.7).

The position of the canine can vary in the mandible in relation to the shape of the arch and, consequently, it is essential to assess the direction of the root, which is often anterior to the crown. In these cases, the X-ray beam should be directed from the mesial aspect of the tooth.

- *Centring point*: along the line of the tooth, as assessed when placing the film into the arch, 1 cm above the lower border of the mandible
- *Angulation*: −20 to −30°
- *Anode-film distance*: 20 cm

(Fig. 5.14)

Key points

Angulation and direction of X-ray-beam Lines of concentration

- mandible — 1 cm above lower border of mandible
- maxilla — ala-tragal line angles of bisection — general guide
- mandible molar 0° — incisors −25°
- maxilla molars 25° — incisors-55

N.B. horizontal angulation vital proclined tooth — increase angulation retroinclined tooth — decrease angulation

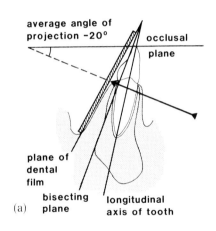

(a)

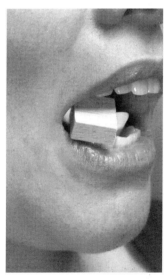

(c)

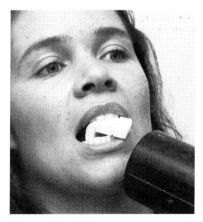

(d)

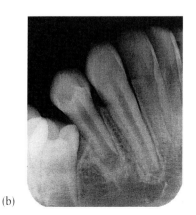

(b)

Fig. 5.14   Lower canine region: (a) the central ray directed at a vertical angle of −20°; (b) the tooth is slightly diagonal on the film; (c) film and holder positioned in the mouth; (d) patient in the vertical position — note that the film and crown are not in contact, in order to keep the film flat.

Lower incisor region

Place the film with the vertical axis obliquely under the tongue, with the crowns in contact, and leaving 5 mm of it above them. Usually, it is possible to obtain diagnostic views of the four incisors on one film, but when there is a very narrow arch, it may be necessary to take two small 2.2 × 3.5 cm intra-oral films behind each central and lateral incisor — adjusting the centring points accordingly.

With the anode–film distance of 20 cm, and film holders, the crown – film distance may be increased and the angle of bisection decreased. This may also be achieved without film holders by putting a cotton wool roll between the tooth and film. (see Fig. 5.15 (d)).

- *Centring point*: midline, 1 cm above the lower border of the mandible
- *Angulation*: −20 to −30°
- *Anode-film distance*: 20 cm

(Fig. 5.15)

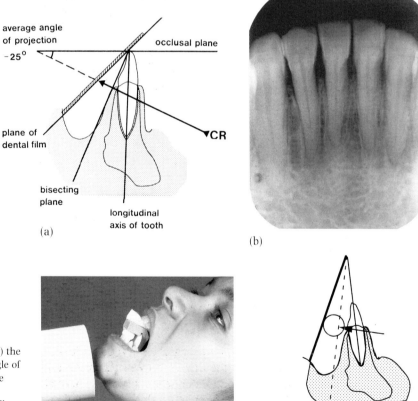

Fig. 5.15   Lower incisor region: (a) the central ray directed at a vertical angle of −25°; (b) the film positioned with the long axis vertical; (c) patient in the working position; (d) cotton wool roll placed between the tooth and film, when a film holder is not used.

In cases of marked protuberance of the chin, it is necessary to adapt the standard technique to prevent the projection of the thickened area around the symphysis menti obscuring the detail round and over the apexes — The centring point may be raised or the chin lowered.

- Where the arch is excessively narrow, it may be necessary to try another technique — parallel film using a small periapical film or the midline oblique occlusal (Fig. 5.16).

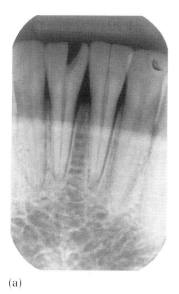

(a)

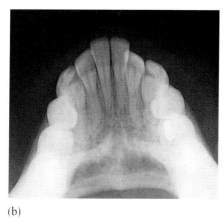

(b)

Fig. 5.16 (a) Small periapical film demonstrating lower central incisors; (b) central midline occlusal.

Upper molar region

The film is placed with the long axis horizontally, behind the molar teeth, leaving 2 mm below the crowns.

- *Centring point*: where the perpendicular 1 cm behind the outer canthus of the eye crosses the ala-tragus line (only when horizontal)
- *Angulation*: 20 to 30°
- *Anode-film distance*: 20 cm

(Fig. 5.17)

- The superimposition of the zygomatic bone, in patients with low palates, is one of the great problems in the bisecting angle technique of this region.

In many cases, a solution can be found by placing the film further into the mouth in order to lessen the angle between the tooth and film. (See Ch. 6 for details of the Long-anode technique.) This necessitates the use of a film holder or, if not available, the placement of one or two cotton wool rolls between the lower border of the film and the palatal surface of the teeth.

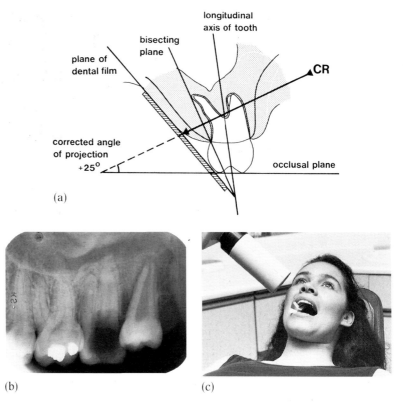

(a)

(b)   (c)

Fig. 5.17   Upper molar region: (a) and (b) the central ray directed at +25°;
(c) patient in the working position.

Ideally, the anode–film distance should be lengthened to compensate for the increased object–film distance and, as there is less angle between the film and tooth, the angle on the X-ray beam may be reduced and directed below the zygoma (Fig. 5.18).

This is the compromise that inevitably evolves between the bisecting angle technique and the parallel film technique. Because even with this latter technique, for example, and its use of filmholders, problems can arise in some mouths.

It may not be possible, to place the film high enough to project the apex on to the film, In this case, one would come back to the bisecting angle technique, taking two projections, each with a different lateral angulation. (These problems are discussed more fully in Chapter 6.)

To demonstrate clearly the three roots of the 6:

1. One view is taken with the X-ray beam directed more acutely from the mesial aspect — in order to throw the zygoma distal to the palatal roots of the first and second molars — and the angu-

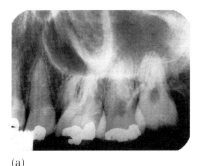
(a)

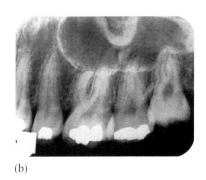
(b)

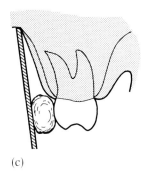
(c)

Fig. 5.18 (a) Directing the beam at 25°, the zygoma may become superimposed over the roots of the 1st molar tooth; (b) use of one or two cotton wool rolls, in order to lower the angle between the tooth and film; (c) this decreases the vertical angle of the central ray from 25° with zygoma superimposed, to 15°.

lation increased to 30 or 35°. Be sure that the film is placed posteriorly enough, as the image of the tooth will be projected distally. The central beam is parallel to the direction of the space between the premolars and the first molar.

2. The second film is taken in the usual lateral direction but the angulation may be lowered to 15–20°, demonstrating the buccal roots. The mesio-buccal root is usually seen in this projection, but the disto-buccal root can be seen in either view, depending upon configuration of the roots.

3. For endodontic procedures, it is sometimes necessary to take a further radiograph with a more acute lateral angulation, or even in the completely opposite direction, with the X-ray beam angled to the crown from the distal aspect (Fig. 5.19).

Third molar
Speed is very important when radiographing this region, as the film causes the patient discomfort due to the sensitivity of the posterior portion of the palate.

The Worth holder can be cery useful in this region. Place the film with 1 cm of the clip just above the lower border, or with the film inclining slightly upward — but be very careful that the film remains flat. If necessary, use a cotton wool wool roll, below the film holder, to achieve a firm bite without curving the film. It is usually helpful to mould the upper anterior corner of the film.

Technique is as for the general view of molar teeth because centring is to the centre of the film, and it is impossible to place the upper third molar in the centre of the film.

If the tooth is unerupted, the central beam angle may need to be increased by 5–10°.

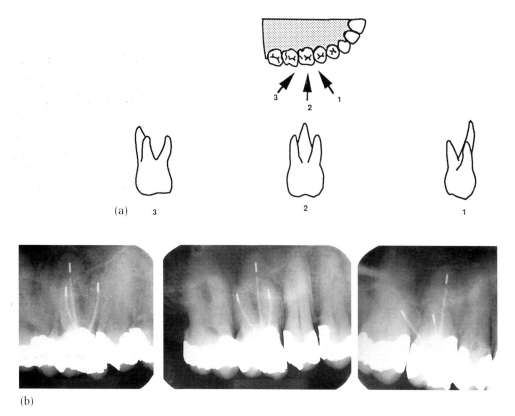

(a)

(b)

Fig. 5.19 (a) Diagrammatic illustration of the 1st upper molar, the X-ray beam coming from three different directions — Direction 1 will also have increased vertical angulation, to throw the zygomatic arch distally, apparently shortening the buccal roots; (b) radiographs to show the practical application of these variations.

Upper premolar region

Place the film with the long axis horizontally, behind the teeth, with 3 mm below the crowns. Care must be taken to place the teeth to the centre of the film, which generally means slight moulding of the upper anterior corner of the film to obtain good object–film contact.

As with the lower premolar region, it is sometimes easier to place the film diagonally in relation to the teeth, incorporating a cotton wool roll to keep the film from curving excessively.

- *Centring point*: where the perpendicular from the midpoint of the infra-orbital margin crosses the line of concentration (ala-tragal line) or above the corner of the mouth
- *Angulation*: 35–40°
- *Anode–film distance*: 20 cm

(Fig. 5.20)

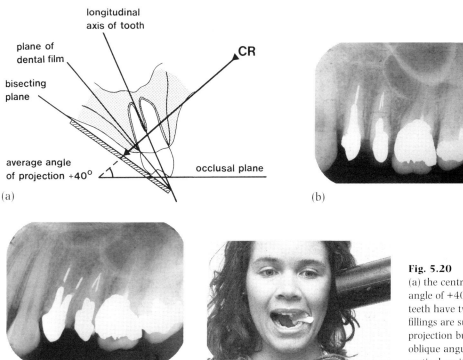

(a)

(b)

(c)

(d)

Fig. 5.20 Upper premolar region: (a) the central ray directed at a vertical angle of +40°; (b) and (c) both premolar teeth have two root canals, and the root fillings are superimposed in the straight projection but separated with a mesial oblique angulation; (d) the patient in the vertical position.

- Due to the soft tissue outline of the cheek, which bears no relationship to the bony contour of the maxilla, it is difficult to assess the horizontal angulation of the X-ray beam.

Care should be taken, when introducing the film into the mouth, to visualize the angulation necessary. In order to separate the two roots of a premolar, it is necessary to exaggerate the lateral angulation and to approach the tooth obliquely. The X-ray beam is directed from the medial aspect parallel to the direction used for the lateral incisor (see Fig. 5.20 (b) and (c)). This is particularly necessary for root canal treatment.

Upper canine region

This is usually the most curved area of the maxilla and, consequently — in order that the film should be flat behind this area, without too much angle between the film and tooth — it is useful to place the film diagonally, behind the long axis of the canine, leaving 3–4 mm below the crown. In a wide arch, this is not necessary, and the film can be placed horizontally, but with the upper anterior corner carefully moulded.

Remember that the root is usually distal to the crown, so allow for the tilt of the tooth. Also, the position of the canine can vary, owing to the shape of the arch, so assess its position when introducing the film into the mouth.

- *Centring point*: the ala of nose along the interdental space between the canine and the first premolar.
- *Angulation*: 45–50°
- *Anode–film distance*: 20 cm

(Fig. 5.21)

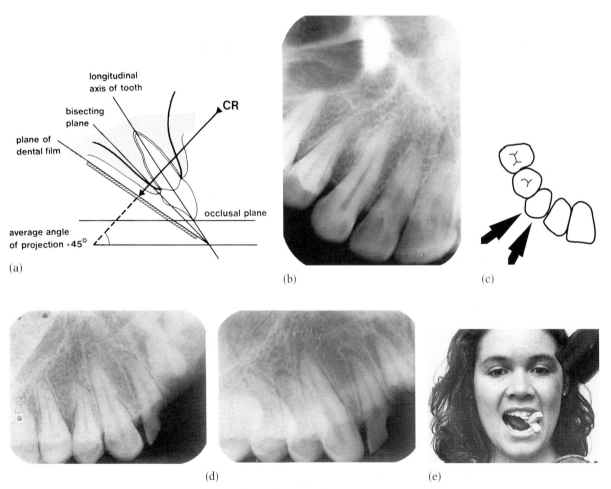

Fig. 5.21 Upper canine region: (a) the central ray directed at a vertical angle of +45°; (b) film placed diagonally, behind the canine; (c) diagram demonstrating the correct lateral angulation between the canine and the first premolar; (d) films demonstrating differences in lateral angulation; (e) patient in the vertical position.

Upper incisor region

In order to be able to separate the roots of the upper incisors per-fectly,an individual film should be taken for each incisor Lateral incisors generally need more angle than central incisors. Practically, a compromise is reached and two films are taken — one for each central and lateral incisor. The central beam is directed along the interdental space between the 1 and 2, remembering the importance of arc of the maxilla, and not the rotation of the teeth within it — thus angling the X-ray beam towards the sagittal plane.

Place the film with the long axis vertical, behind the tooth or teeth to be examined, leaving 3 mm below the crowns. The narrowness of the arch can tend to keep the film flat – almost horizontal in some cases (Fig. 5.22).

- *Centring point*: along the vertical axis of the tooth, through the nose, to the extension of the ala-tragal line in the incisor region
- *Angulation*: 50–60° (average 50°)
- *Anode–film distance*: 20 cm.

The angulation for the central incisors will vary more than for any other tooth in the mouth:

1. Very retroclined teeth will need only 40°. (Below this, the angle of incidence will cause distortion of the surrounding tissues, but may be lowered when only the length of the root canal is required).

2. In proclined teeth, the angle may need to be increased to 60–65°

(The variation of maxillary anatomy is discussed further in Chapter 6.)

Children
In very young children, when the deciduous teeth are to be examined, place the intra-oral dental film with the long axis horizontally, behind the teeth in the occlusal plane, and with the patient biting on to the film.

- *Centring point*: in the midline, down to the line of concentration.
- *Angulation*: 60°.
- *Anode–film distance*: 20 cm.
(see Fig. 5.22 (g))

Comprehensive survey

If a comprehensive survey of the teeth is to be undertaken, 15 films are necessary. This includes one for each region of the mouth (incisor, canine, premolar, and molar), with an additional film in the upper incisor region, as it is normally difficult to demonstrate these four teeth on one periapical film. The lateral incisor may sometimes be

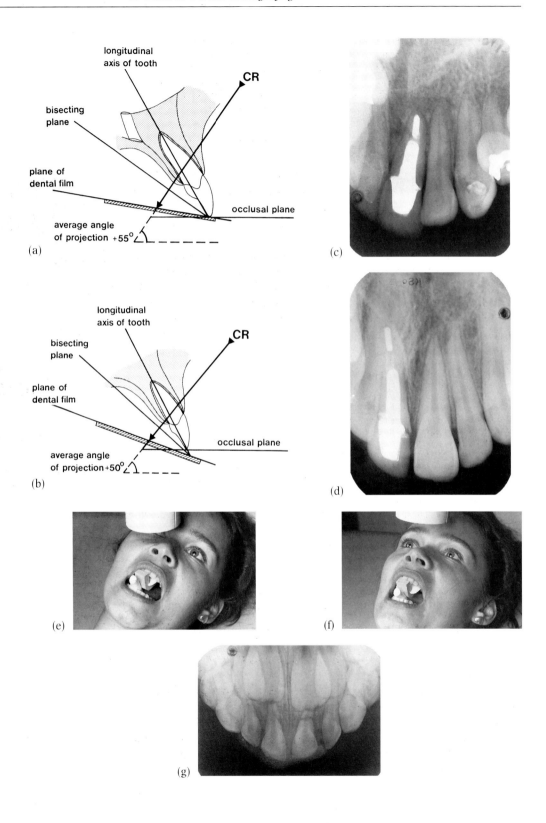

(a)

longitudinal axis of tooth

CR

bisecting plane

plane of dental film

occlusal plane

average angle of projection +55°

(b)

longitudinal axis of tooth

CR

bisecting plane

plane of dental film

occlusal plane

average angle of projection +50°

(c)

(d)

(e)

(f)

(g)

Fig. 5.22 Upper incisor region: (a) lateral incisor — the central ray directed at a vertical angle of +55°; (b) central incisor region — the central ray directed at a vertical angle of about +50°; (c) film of lateral incisor; (d) film of central incisor; (e) and (f) patient in the working position — demonstrating the differing positions of the film and the X-ray beam for the left incisor region and the midline, by rotating the head towards the X-ray beam; (g) film in occlusal plane, demonstrating fractured a|a in a 3-year-old child.

assessed with the canine. Some clinicians will compromise with 10 or 11 films for an overall survey – this may be adequate, but not complete.

Today, awareness of radiation dosage has become very important for the dentist and patient: the ALARA principle is to be encouraged. Many dental practitioners have, or have access to, rotational panoramic apparatus which will give an overall scan. This reduces the necessity for comprehensive radiographs of all the teeth to be taken routinely. Instead, this overall scan only needs supplementing with individual radiographs for problematic areas. Nevertheless, there is no substitute for the detail and accuracy of good periapical radiography (Fig. 5.23).

5.2   PARALLAX

Parallax is a technique for ascertaining the relative position of two objects. The easiest way to visualize this is to put the forefingers of both hands, one in front of the other, level with your eyes.

Move the head one way and then the other way, without altering the position of your fingers.

The finger furthest away will move with the head, the nearer one will move in the opposite direction.

This is the action of the X-ray tube in relation to two objects (Fig. 5.24).

Parallax is used primarily for ascertaining the position of retained roots, unerupted teeth, and foreign bodies. In practice, two exposures are made. The position of the film should be similar in each case, with enough lateral movement to allow for the exaggerated projection of the image.

The vertical angulation of the X-ray beam and the centring point remain constant.

The only variant is the horizontal angulation, which should swing through about 40° (Fig. 5.25).

The other application of parallax is in the separation of root canals of upper molar teeth. Here, the situation is reversed — the position of the roots is known, but the shift is used to prevent superimposition (see Fig. 5.19).

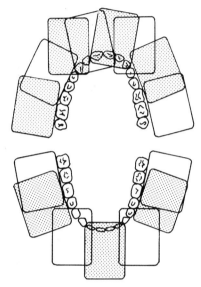

Fig. 5.23   Fifteen dental films are used for a full, all-round intra-oral examination — eight films in the upper jaw and seven films in the lower jaw.

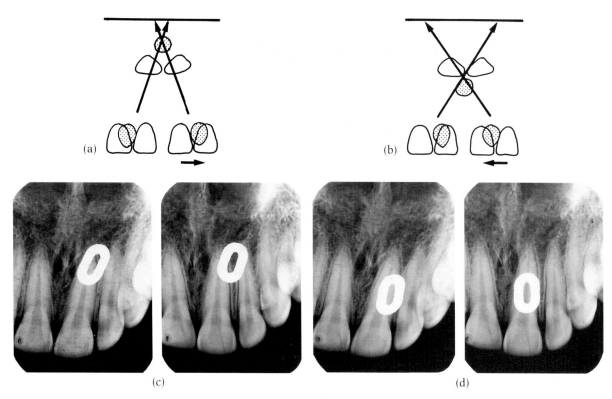

(a)   (b)

(c)   (d)

Fig. 5.24   Diagrammatic representation of parallax in the upper incisor region: (a) palatal shift; (b) buccal shift. Radiographs on a dry skull demonstrating: (c) palatal shift; (d) buccal shift.

Fig. 5.25   Parallax films showing an unerupted supernumerary in right incisor region. The supernumerary lies palatal to the unerupted right central incisor.

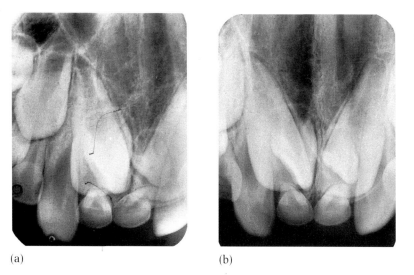

(a)   (b)

Parallax is not limited to the horizontal plane, but may also be applied to the vertical plane, for example, between bisecting angle periapical views and bitewings. It may also be observed between dental panoramic tomographs and intra-oral views — periapical or occlusals.

Care must be taken when observing shifts between intra and extra-oral views — remember that the X-ray beam approaches the teeth from the opposite aspect. Prior knowledge of the pattern of the X-ray beam scan, in a particular apparatus, is essential.

REFERENCES AND FURTHER READING

Waite, E. (1996). *Essentials of dental radiography and radiology* (2nd edn). Churchill Livingstone.

Haring, J.L. and Lind, L.J. (1996). Dental radiography: principles and techniques. W.B. Saunders and Co.

Fox, N.A., Fletcher, G.A., and Horner, K. (1995). Localising maxillary canines using dental panoramic tomography. *British Dental Journal*

Frommer, H.H. (1987). *Radiology for dental auxiliaries* (4th edn). C.V. Mosby, St Louis.

Goaz, P.W. and White, S.C. (1987). *Oral radiology — principles and interpretation* (2nd edn). C.V. Mosby, St Louis.

Manson-Hing, L.R. (1985). *Fundamentals of dental radiography* (2nd edn). Lea and Febiger, Philadelphia.

Perlman, C. (1973). *A student guide to dental radiology.* The University of Texas Dental Branch, Houston.

Updegrave, W.J. (1971). *New horizons in periapical and interproximal radiography.* Rinn Corporation, Illinois.

Wiessman, D.D. (1973). *Manual of rectangular field collimation for intra-oral periapical radiography.* The University of California at Los Angeles.

Rinn Corporation. *Intra-oral radiography with Rinn XCP/BIA instruments.* Rinn Corporation, Illinois.

NRPB. (1994). *Guidelines on radiology standards for primary dental care.*

ICRP. (1985). *Approved Code of Practice. The protection of persons against ionising radiation arising from any work activity. The Ionising Radiation Regulations.* HMSO, London.

6 Comparison of the different intra-oral radiographic techniques

6.1 INTRODUCTION

It is worthwhile considering the advantages and disadvantages of intra-oral periapical techniques, and when each one is applicable, since **Inappropriate techniques** can misrepresent pathology. (Fig. 6.1)

If all dental X-ray apparatus were the same — preferably with a 40 cm anode–film distance — and all mouths had anatomically identical dental arches, then the Paralleling intra-oral technique would be the obvious choice.

This would also presume that all the operators, dentists, dental auxiliaries, and radiographers had had comprehensive theoretical and practical training, and that there was adequate funding **for equipment**. Unfortunately, this is not so — consequently, we must look at the problems we encounter in the real world.

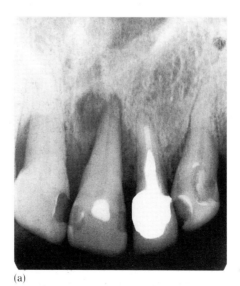 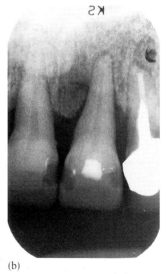

Fig. 6.1 Intra-oral periapical films showing the movement of a radiolucent area on the mesial side of the apex; (a) with the bisecting angle technique, radiolucency appears to be at the apex; (b) with the paralleling technique, the translucency is at the crest of the bone and extends all the way to the apex.

(a)   (b)

Firstly, however, let us remember the objective — perfect radiographic representation of teeth — before we consider the difficulties. The principles for an ideal radiograph are:-

- the object and film should be parallel
- the object – film distance should be minimal
- the X-ray beam should be at 90° to the object and film
- the X-ray beam should be parallel.

6.2 BASIC ANATOMICAL PROBLEMS OF THE DENTAL ARCHES AND TEETH

There is an enormous range of *normal* anatomy within the dental arches. This presents problems when undertaking intra-oral radiography, whichever technique is chosen.

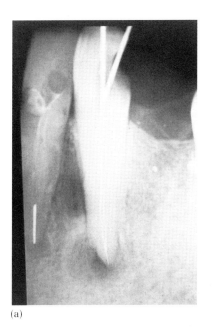
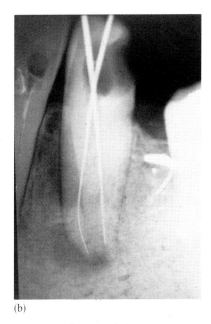
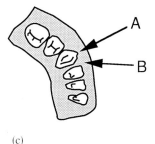

(a)   (b)   (c)

Fig. 6.2   (a) and (b) Lower canine demonstrating two roots during endodontic treatment; (c) the horizontal angulation necessary to separate the roots, from the mesial aspect.

6.2.1 The mandible

1. The relationship of the film to the tooth, when positioning it in the mouth, is restricted by the depth of the floor of the mouth.

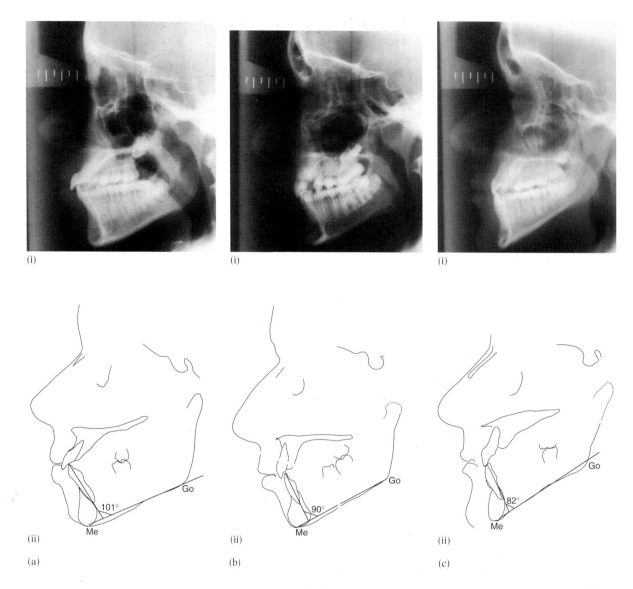

Fig. 6.3 Normal varients in inclination of mandibular incisors in relation to the mandilular (Menton–Gorion): (a) proclined — (i) cephalometric lateral facial bones (ii) tracing; (b) average — (i) cephalometric lateral facial bones (ii) tracing; (c) retroclined — (i) cephalometric lateral facial bones (ii) tracing.

This is determined by the location of the mylohyoid muscle in relation to the lingual surface of the mandible, that is, the angulation necessary to keep the film flat and as near to the teeth under examination as possible.

2. Mandibular tori — bony exostoses on the lingual surface of the mandible — prevent close association of the film to the teeth and, sometimes, the angulation of the incisors (see Fig. 6.5).

3. The long axes of the lower premolar teeth are proclined relative to the lingual plate of the alveolar process.

4. The long axes of the mandibular third molars are distally inclined at 25°, and proclined at 25°.

5. The lower canine occasionally has two roots — buccal and lingual —, necessitating adjustment of the horizontal angulation if separation is required (Fig. 6.2).

6. The average lower incisors are at ± 92° to the mandibular line (Fig. 6.3).

6.2.2 The maxilla

1. Placement of the film is dependent upon the shape and height of the palate:
   (a) Shallow palates do not allow the film to be parallel to the apexes; high vaulted palates do not present this problem.
   (b) In high vaulted palates, the problem may occur in the canine region as the arch narrows anteriorly.

2. A maxillary torus may have the same limitations as the shallow palate.

3. These limitations are of greater significance when the apexes of the teeth are in the maxillary antrum.

4. The maxillary canine is slightly retroclined (20°) in relation to the palatal alveolar plate.

5. The maxillary first premolar has two roots — the buccal and the palatal. Again, if separation is required, there will need to be adjustment to the horizontal angulation of the X-ray beam. (See Fig. 5.20 (c) and (d), p. 97).

6. The long axis of the upper canine is at 15° to the vertical, when viewed buccally, inclining towards the first premolar.

7. The average inclination of the upper maxillary incisor is ± 108° to the maxillary line.

8. Inclinations of the teeth vary and must be accounted for. This is why a standard technique with film holders is so important, in order to adjust the angulation to compensate for the original shortening or elongation.

9. In a Class II, division 1 malocclusion, the upper central incisors are proclined and will need more than average angulation. In a class II, division 2 malocclusion, the upper central incisors are

retro clined and need less than average angulation. Care must be taken in these cases because the bisecting angle technique has a limit to the amount of reduction of angulation possible, without distorting the trabeculation. The paralleling technique will tend to foreshorten the tooth (Fig. 6.4).

10. The upper molars have three roots and to distinguish each buccal root from the palatal root, horizontal angulation of the X-ray beam must again be adjusted (See Fig 5.19).

11. A pronounced maxillary tuberosity will compromise parallelism.

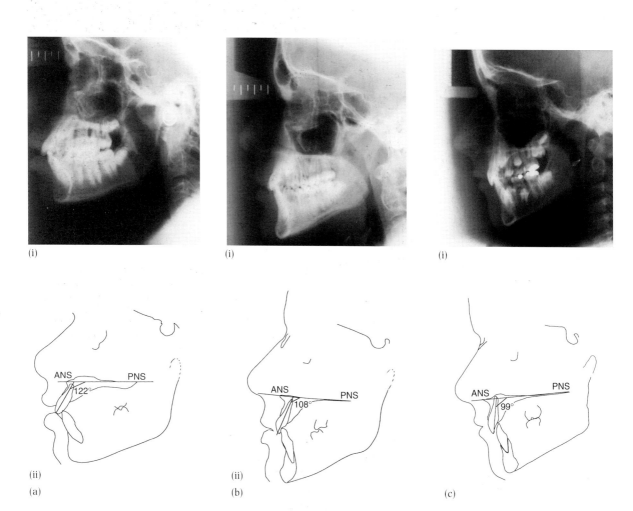

Fig. 6.4 Normal varients in inclination of maxillary incisors in relation to the maxillary line (anterior nasal spine–posterior nasal spine): (a) proclined — (i) cephalometric lateral facial bones (ii) tracing; (b) average — (i) cephalometric lateral facial bones (ii) tracing; (c) retroclined — (i) cephalometric lateral facial bones (ii) tracing.

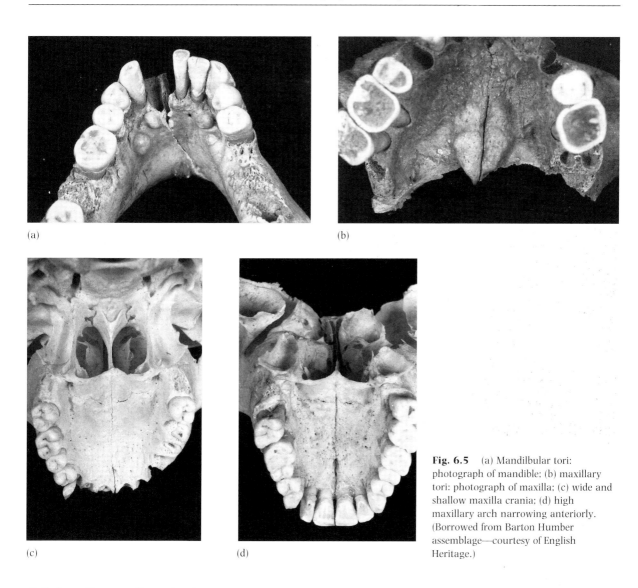

(a)

(b)

(c)

(d)

Fig. 6.5 (a) Mandilbular tori: photograph of mandible; (b) maxillary tori: photograph of maxilla; (c) wide and shallow maxilla crania; (d) high maxillary arch narrowing anteriorly. (Borrowed from Barton Humber assemblage—courtesy of English Heritage.)

6.2.3 General variations

1. The dental arches are in the form of catenary curves: one behind the canines — a straight line connecting the distal of the canine to the mesiobuccal cusp of the first molar — and, another, a final straight line from the mesiobuccal of the first molar to the distal of the third molar. There is little variation in this basic shape and means that a maximum of three teeth can be taken on any one film.

2. Crowding of teeth may cause some superimposition, requiring readjustment of the intra-oral technique.

Key points

Anatomical variations which cause differences in the tooth-film relationship

1. Mandible
   - depth of the floor of the mouth
   - location of mylohyoid muscle
   - mandibular tori
   - inclination of teeth to lingual plate
2. Maxilla
   - height and shape of the palate
   - maxillary tori
   - relationship of the palatal alveolar plate
   - inclination of upper maxillary incisors
3. Rotation of teeth within the alveolus

3. Again, rotation of teeth must be taken into account when assessing the choice of periapical radiographic techniques.
4. With the paralleling technique, even if the film and alveolar process are parallel, the accuracy of the projection will be dependent upon the angulation of the tooth within it.
5. With the bisecting angle technique, variation is allowed for — but not always assessed correctly.

6.3   PARALLELING FILM TECHNIQUE

6.3.1   Advantages

1. It should project a true lateral image of the long axis of the tooth.
2. The alveolar crest is demonstrated in its true relationship to the teeth.
3. There is no superimposition of the zygomatic buttress of the maxilla over the upper molar roots.
4. The patient can be placed in any comfortable position — horizontally or vertically — suitable to the operator and the mobility of the tube head.
5. The film is flat, as film holders are essential to position and maintain the film in the mouth. Thus, There will be less likelihood of distortion due to curvature of the film.
6. With an anode–object distance of 40 cm, there is minimal enlargement and, consequently, optimum definition.
7. It necessitates a longer anode-film distance. Consequently, the higher kilovoltage needed will reduce the radiation skin dosage.
8. As long as the technique is accurately carried out, it is easier to achieve reproducible results.

6.3.2   Disadvantages

1. This procedure needs careful and accurate placement of the film in the oral cavity. If the tooth and film are not parallel, the true object of the technique will be lost.
2. It is difficult to achieve separation of roots with a lateral angulation adjustment of the X-ray beam.
3. More films need to be taken for a comprehensive diagnosis, particularly in the incisor and canine region.

4. In many instances, more extensive diagnostic information is required, around and beyond the apex, than can be demonstrated in this precise technique.

5. The film holders, in keeping the film flat, often cause discomfort. This means that if the patient does not bite down fully, the apex is not demonstrated.

6. The necessity to use film holders makes the technique impractical, without modification, during an endodontic procedure, where comparative views are essential. (Though there are now adapted endodontic film holders coming on to the market. For example, see Fig. 6.9).

7. It is more time-consuming, than the bisecting angle technique.

8. Therefore, it is questionable whether it is suitable for younger children.

6.4   BISECTING ANGLE TECHNIQUE

6.4.1   Advantages

(The authors wish to emphasize that they have always used and recommended the use of film holders in this technique)

1. The introduction of the film into the mouth is easier for the patient. It does not need elaborate film holders — simple ones help the patient to keep still (see Fig. 5.6 (a) and (b), p. 84).

2. The film can be adapted to the shape of most dental arches.

3. More teeth may be demonstrated on one film, without overlap. Standard films can nearly always be used.

4. The area beyond the apex and unerupted teeth can be demonstrated.

5. It is easily adaptable for endodontic treatment.

6. Satisfactory results are possible at 20 cm anode–object distance.

7. It can be undertaken speedily for difficult patients or those in pain. Though speed is, of course, achieved with experience and consequent competence.

6.4.2   Disadvantages

1. The projection of the tooth gives an oblique image.

2. The loss of bone, or pathology at the alveolar margin, is misrepresented.

3. The technique is often difficult to understand.

4. Accurate comparative work needs standard parameters including, possibly, even the same operator (though this would likely be the case in general dental practice). So, it is not always so easy to get reproducible results.

6.5   THE LONG ANODE–FILM PERIAPICAL TECHNIQUE

Key points

Long anode–film technique
1. Use film holder to allow for a wider tooth–film distance
2. Angulation of film to tooth, 5–15°
3. Film, flat
4. Horizontal angulation, very important
5. Keep to circular POPUMET field of radiation (diameter box)
6. **Bisect angle between film and teeth**

Key points

Long anode–film technique
1. Disadvantage — some foreshortening of the tooth image
2. Still better than an inaccurate paralleling projection which involves making an angle between the tooth and film without altering the angle of the X-ray beam
3. Dentist, aware of compromise, views film accordingly

When neither of the two more standard techniques are possible or appropriate, the long anode–film periapical technique offers a compromise.

1. The film is placed into the mouth using a film holder with a longer biting projection — perhaps using the paralleling film holder without the collimating attachment (See Fig. 4.12(e), p. 68.)

2. The film should make an angle of 5–15° to the tooth. Consequently, the crown will not be parallel to the film which must remain flat.

3. The object–film distance will be increased, as is necessary with the paralleling technique.

4. It is still very important that the lateral angulation should be correctly assessed to prevent overlapping of teeth, as in all other intra-oral periapical techniques. (See Fig. 4.5) If the paralleling holder is used, the arm of the holder helps to assess the lateral angulation, being in line with the area under examination.

5. The anode-film distance should be appropriate to the collimating device keeping to the POPUMET regulations (Protection for Persons Undergoing Medical Examination or Treatment).

6. The X-ray beam should bisect the angle between the film and teeth. The arm of the paralleling holder, if used, will help to define the position of the film.

7. This bisecting angle between the tooth and film will be considerabley lower than with the conventional bisecting angle technique.

8. This technique will not foreshorten the tooth as much as if the paralleling situation cannot be met, and the X-ray beam is still directed at 90° to the film (Fig. 6.6).

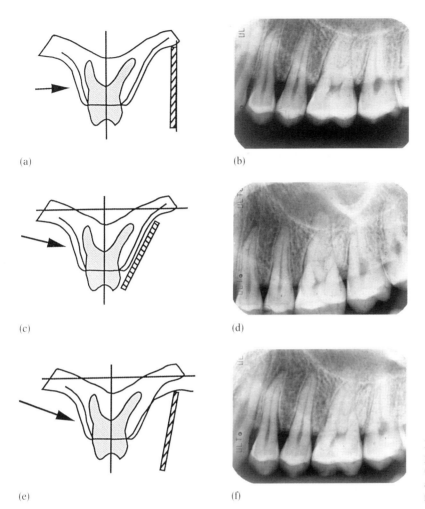

(a)

(b)

(c)

(d)

(e)

(f)

Fig. 6.6 Diagrams and film: (a) and (b) projection as for paralleling technique; (c) and (d) projection as for bisecting angle technique; (e) and (f) projection as for long anode film technique.

6.5.1 Differences from the paralleling technique

1. The relationship between the apex and the film will remain almost constant, but the crown–film distance is less than the apex–film distance.

2. This compromise position of the film holder and tooth can best be undertaken with a 40 cm anode–collimating device. Nevertheless, as with the paralleling technique, it is perfectly adequate at the 20 cm anode–film distance.

3. There will be some foreshortening of the teeth.

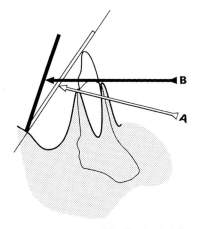

Fig. 6.7 Position of the film for (A) the bisecting angle technique; (B) the compromise long-anode technique.

6.5.2   Differences from the bisecting angle technique

1. The distance between the crown and the film is increased, for example, as demonstrated for the lower incisor teeth (Fig. 6.7).
2. It allows the angle of bisection to be considerably lessened.
3. Compromise image is more accurate.
4. There may be some lessening of detail periapically if the anode distance is 20 cm, due to the increased object–film distance. Results will be better with the 40 cm distance.

6.6   GENERAL CONSIDERATIONS REGARDING CHOICE OF TECHNIQUE

1. The intra-oral paralleling technique can be undertaken with an anode–object distance of 40 or 20 cm. Though 40 cm is the ideal anode–object distance, 20 cm is the more practical distance in general practice and entails minimal enlargement and loss of quality (See Fig. 4.10, p. 66.)
2. Apparatus with a fixed output of 60–75 kVp gives an adequate quality X-ray beam for the paralleling technique. Obviously, the higher the kVp then the better the definition, the lower the radiation skin dosage, and shorter the exposure time. The time taken to position the X-ray tube and return the exposure activator is longer than the actual exposure time, so the ease of undertaking any technique is of paramount importance.
3. In practice, there are many situations where a compromise is arrived at naturally between the bisecting and the paralleling intra-oral techniques — that is, the long anode–film periapical technique. This technique is an obvious choice, for example, when the dental arches are not able to accommodate the true paralleling situation.
4. Ideally, if comparable radiographs are all-important, then either one of the more conventional techniques is simpler to standardize.
5. The choice of techniques depends upon the degree of patient co-operation. When this is not forthcoming, for example, when the patient is in pain, then speed – usually combined with the necessity to include the apical area — becomes essential.
6. It is easier for the dental undergraduate to be taught the two distinct, conventional intra-oral techniques, for it is only with experience that the compromise technique can be satisfactorily assessed and undertaken.

7. During the clinical examination, the dentist should assess the technique to be undertaken with regard to which will give the most accurate image of the information required.

8. The dentist must be aware of the differences in the image projection with either conventional technique or the compromise.

    - Dental Radiography is an area in dentistry where a very good understanding of anatomy is essential in order to be able to make the necessary adjustment when viewing the radiographs and to take this into account, for a correct diagnosis.
    - Many dentists, with this knowledge, use the paralleling periapical technique, together with appropriate film holders and, as a very useful 'aiming' device, collimators. They are aware of the foreshortening factor and allow for this.

9. Cost is always a factor for the dentist in general practice. The higher kilovoltage apparatus necessary for the 40 cm anode distance is more expensive, plus, investment in paralleling film holders is needed.

10. Keeping up to date with dental radiography is, of course, to be encouraged — as the 1994 Guidelines on Radiology Standards for Primary Dental Care state.

The choice of technique is dependent upon:

- area of the mouth, with its anatomical limitations
- particular area of interest within the tooth.

6.6.1 Anatomical factors contributing to choice of intra-oral technique

For each dental region, use of the following techniques is recommended:

(1) lower molars — dependent upon the depth of the mouth and object–film distance, but usually parallel film technique, although the longer anode–film distance is less advantageous because tooth and film are in contact;

(2) lower premolars — dependent upon the depth of the floor of the mouth and object–film distance, parallel film technique, even with 20 cm anode distance;

(3) lower canine — Long anode-film technique in most cases, because the position of the film in relation to the tooth is vital and compromise necessary;

(4) lower incisor — long anode-film technique (bisecting angle technique involves too large an angle between tooth and film and parallel film technique is anatomically difficult); see Fig. 6.7

Key points

Suggested choice of periapical technique Mandible
1. Molar — parallel film, 20 cm
2. Premolar — parallel film
3. Canine — long anode-film, tooth film relationship vital
4. Incisor — long anode-film, dependent on area of interest

Maxilla
1. Molar — long anode-film or parallel film if anatomically possible
2. Premolar — long anode-film or parallel film if anatomically possible
3. Canine — long anode-film, film oblique (periapical — Bisecting angle)
4. Incisor — parallel film with narrow film or long anode-film (periapical — bisecting angle)

(5) upper molars — parallel film technique in high arches; long anode-film technique in flatter arches;

(6) upper premolars — as upper molars;

(7) upper canine — long anode-film technique, with film obliquely positioned (parallel film technique very difficult to achieve and bisecting angle technique foreshortens but clear around the apex);

(8) upper incisors — parallel film technique with small paedadontic films for periodontal assessment bisecting angle technique for apexes, long anode-film technique for overall assessment.

6.6.2   General rules for a particular area of interest within the tooth

For each of the given areas, use of the following techniques is recommended:

(1) the apex, for example, apical pathology — bisecting angle technique;

(2) alveolar crest, to assess bone loss over a period of time, which is needs comparative imaging projections — accurate parallel film technique centred over the alveolar crest, possibly with a cotton wool roll placed below the crowns, or vertical bitewings;

(3) alveolar crest and entire tooth, for example, root resorption — parallel film technique, or possibly long anode-film technique;

(4) area beyond the apex and unerupted teeth — bisecting angle technique, progressing to the oblique occlusal;

(5) endodontic diagnosis and treatment — as appropriate, preferably using a film holder (either one on the market or own adaptation) (See Figs 6.9 and 6.10).

Exposure factors

Where the exposure times are preset for different areas of the mouth, be careful to take into account the differences between the paralleling and bisecting angle techniques. Check for which technique the exposures are set. If the apparatus offers an option of a longer 30–40 cm collimating device, then remember to increase the exposure factors — bear in mind that even if the anode distance is the same, the density of bone will vary (Fig. 6.8).

Finally, variations in individual patients' skeletal patterns and differences between ethnic groups will always create problems in intra-oral periapical radiography.

If it were simple there would be no choice.

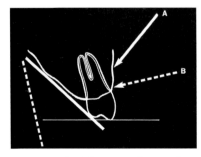

Fig. 6.8 The difference in density of bone in the premolar region for (a) the bisecting angle technique and (b) the paralleling technique.

6.7 COMPARISON OF VERTICAL AND WORKING POSITION FOR PERIAPICAL RADIOGRAPHY

6.7.1 Advantages of the vertical position

1. A part from during endodontic procedures, most diagnostic routine radiographs are taken at the beginning or the end of the appointment.

2. Dental auxiliaries are being trained to take dental radiographs and, consequently, play a positive part in making the practice cost effective. Therefore, the patient will leave the dentist's surgery and move into another room dedicated to radiography.

3. X-ray apparatus and the upright chair occupies less space.

4. Radiographically, this is a more efficient position; standard techniques can be quickly and easily undertaken; anatomical landmarks are clearly visible; baselines can be set; and the position of the tube can be viewed objectively from both aspects.

5. Traditionally, dental radiology departments have worked with the patient sitting upright.

6. In X-ray departments, or large group practices with a separate X-ray room, the time and motion principle can be more readily applied.

7. Consequently, dental undergraduates, dental auxiliaries, and, of course, radiographers, are taught with the chair upright.

8. This may feel more comfortable and secure for the nervous patient.

6.7.2 Advantages of the dental working position

1. Dentists are now accustomed to assessing their patient's teeth in this position and, certainly during treatment, it will cause the least disturbance to the patient and to surgery procedure.

2. The use of film holders with centring devices will overcome the problem of reorientating the baseline and tube.

3. Less radiation dosage will be given to the abdomen when radiographing the upper incisor region.

4. It prevents an easy error that when the dental working chair is moved vertically, it will not be to the full 90 degrees, so care must then be taken that the occlusal plane is adjusted into the horizontal.

6.8   TIME AND MOTION PROCEDURE

When considering any individual intra-oral technique, a few general rules on procedure may be helpful:

1.   Explain to the patient about the procedure being undertaken.

2.   If used, place the lead rubber (Pastolead) apron on the patient.

3.   Examine the patient's mouth for any deviations from the normal. These may require some adjustment of the standard radiographic techniques.

4.   Remove from the patient anything that will impede the placement of the intra-oral film, or that will cast a radio-opaque shadow upon it, for example, dentures, removable orthodontic appliances, and spectacles.

5.   Set the exposure factors. In most cases this will only mean adjusting the exposure time, but sometimes it may also involve kilovoltage selection. If there is a choice of milliamperage, then pick the one that is suitable to that intra-oral technique, taking the time factor into account.

6.   If possible, set the appropriate angle on the X-ray tube for the tooth or teeth to be examined — at least bring the X-ray tube head adjacent to the area.

7.   Adjust the head-rest or the back of the chair in order that the patient's head can be correctly positioned and immobilized — If necessary, incorporate foam pads.

8.   Place the film into the patient's mouth, with the embossed dot towards the crowns, into whichever position the technique demands but, in all cases, remember that curvature produces distortion. Immobilize the film — with film holders if at all possible — or, in difficult situations, with the patient's finger or by occlusion.

     The actual placement of the film in the patient's mouth should be almost the last act in the taking of a radiograph. This will enable the operator to gain the maximum co-operation from the patient, particularly if the film causes any discomfort

9.   Check the position of the patient's head in the vertical and horizontal planes.

10. Centre the tube head, remembering to assess the direction of the central ray from two aspects, at right angles to each other

11. The operator must stand either 1.5–2.0 m away, at right angles to the X-ray tube head, or behind a lead screen, preferably in a position where the patient can be seen. If constant watch is kept on the patient, between positioning and exposing, many errors, due to movement of the patient's head or the film itself, can be avoided. (See Fig. 1.6, p. 13.)

12. Place a finger on the timing device and hold until the exposure is complete — timers automatically cut out).

13. Remove the film from the patient's mouth and dry it, to prevent any saliva seeping into the packet and, thus, causing a film fault. Special care must be taken to put infection control methods in place.

14. Identify the films clearly for processing. This is especially important if several patients' films are processed at the same time.

15. In the case of automatic processing, some sure means of identification must be used, for example, a small envelope with the patient's name on it.

16. For wet processing, it is helpful to place the films on a dental hanger, with the patient's name clearly marked. This can also be helpful for the eventual viewing and mounting of the films.

17. If used, remove the lead apron from the patient and return it carefully to a position where it is not bent, to prevent the lead from cracking and losing its protective property.

6.9   ECONOMIC CONSIDERATIONS

The initial investment in contemporary apparatus Ionising Radiation Regulations (IRR) of and accessories is significant. Nevertheless, abiding by the 1985 and 1988, with regard to adequate training of the operator, will mean that the diagnostic quality of the radiographs should improve. Suitable quality assurance (see Chapter 16) will also pinpoint problems and help to maintain a high standard of processing. (Processing has, as previously stated, been one of the areas of inadequacy in dental radiography.)

● Altogether, all this, combined with the dentist's judgement upon the suitability of which periapical technique to prescribe and view, should avoid the need for retakes. So, in the long run, the investment will save money (as the 1994 Guidelines imply).

6.10   CONSIDERATIONS FOR ENDODONTIC PROCEDURES

Before treatment is undertaken, it is essential to have control radiographs, but important to remember that these can be give only limited information. In particular, it is difficult to assess the curvature of a root in the bucco-lingual plane, or to identify the relationships of superimposed structures.

Key points

1. Advantages of the vertical position
   — taken at end of appointment so maybe taken by Dental Auixiliary
   — occupies less space
   — easy to standardise radiographic techniques
   — good teaching position
2. Advantages of the working position
   — easy for dentist with film holders
   — less disturbance for patient
   — may give less radiation
3. Time and motion
   — maintains radiographic standards
   — Co-operation of patient

Key points

1. Take control radiographs
2. Assess vertical angulation
   — to include apex
3. In multi-rooted tooth assess horizontal angulation
4. Use *Endodontic procedure* film holders, if at all possible
5. Choose exposure factors to highlight apex and root canal
6. Edge of film, apical to crown

1. Work out the vertical angulation, remembering to centre over the apex, 1 cm apical to the usual centring points. Often, the object–film distance is, of necessity, increased and the consequent enlargement, with lack of definition, can be lessened by increasing the anode–film distance proportionately. If the arches are deep, so that the film and tooth can approach the parallel position, then an adaptation of the paralleling technique may be employed (see Fig. 6.6(e)). If this is impossible, the bisecting angle technique must be used, necessitating on increased angle between the tooth and film.

It is better to get the apex slightly foreshortened than too long, with the consequent possibility of missing it altogether. As previously stated, with knowledge of anatomy, the foreshortening of the image can be disregarded in endodontics (as long as a file has been inserted and radiographed as a control).

2. The lateral angle may be very important in multi-rooted teeth and more than one projection is necessary. Parallax rules apply — the lingual or palatal roots moving with the tube position, and the buccal roots moving in the opposite direction. With extreme lateral angulation — as indicated in some areas, to separate roots — some periapical bony detail must be sacrificed to achieve this effect (Fig. 6.9c).

3. Because of the greater depth of overlying bone, exposure factors should be increased with acute lateral angulation. The exposure factors are also increased when the anode–film–object distance is increased in the paralleling technique.

4. In some teeth, the root can be demonstrated more clearly when the density between the dentine and the canal is more marked. This contrast will be affected if the kilovoltage can be decreased. Remember, however, to increase the milliamperage seconds to compensate for the decreased penetration: 70 kVp, 2.5 mAs; 60 kVp, 5.0 mAs.

Faster films may be used to reduce the radiation exposure.

Whilst this procedure will increase skin dosage, this is preferable to making multiple exposures without useful diagnostic information. The facility to enhance the image is one of the advantages of the digitized image (see Chapter 7).

5. The position of the film is very important: it must remain flat. It can be placed either side of the rubber dam — whichever makes it easier to put the film in the most advantageous position in relation to the apex of the tooth. For upper incisors, the film is often in the occlusal plane.

The use of cotton wool rolls can help to keep the film flat or to achieve a more parallel position, although There are now film holders especially designed for endodontic procedures (Fig. 6.9(a)). It is also

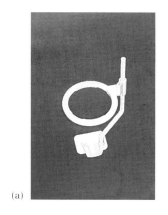
(a)

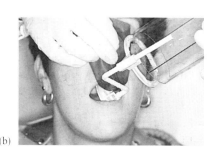
(b)

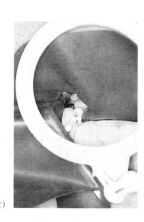
(c)

Fig. 6.9 (a) Film holder for use in endodontics; (b) Endo-rinn; endo-rinn holder with film being positioned in the mouth for ⌊4; (c) the two files, in place, ready for radiographic control film; (d) periapical film, with the mesial oblique projection demonstrating points positioned into the buccal and palatal roots of an ⌊4; (e) Radiograph taken with the exaggerated mesial lateral angulation to separate the roots in a lower molar during root canal treatment.

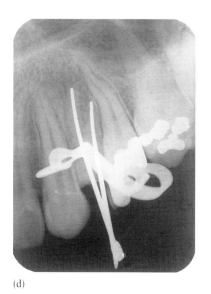

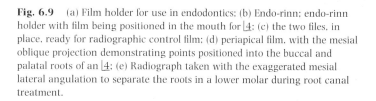

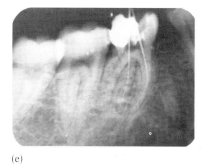

(d)

(e)

possible to adapt a film holder, specially for such use, by adding greenstick composition to the biting surface of the opposing tooth or teeth. The impression made will ensure exact replacement of the film during the endodontic procedure (Fig. 6.10).

Obviously, there is little use in putting the handle, and not the tip, of the file on to the control radiograph. So, in most cases, place the edge of the film apical to the handle of the reamer — in fact, as with other intra-oral films, just apical to the crowns of the teeth.

6. Remember exactly how each projection was taken, so that the necessary alteration in either the vertical or the horizontal angulation

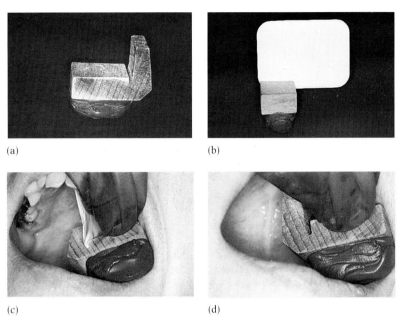

(a)   (b)

(c)   (d)

Fig. 6.10   (a) and (b) Film holder adapted for endodontic procedure by the addition of
a greenstick composition to the biting surface of the opposing, but more mesial, tooth
— the impression so made, in a preoperative exposure, will enable future films to be
repeated in an exactly comparable position; (c) patient with rubber dam and adapted
film holder being positioned in mouth; (d) patient with the holder and film in position.

may be made to improve the image of the apex or apexes for treatment. (See Fig. 6.9 (b) and (c).)

During endodontic procedures it is particularly important to
observe the cross infection recommendations.

6.11   SAFETY FROM CROSS-INFECTION IN RADIOGRAPHY

There is very little evidence for the spread of viral infections from
uncontaminated human saliva, but it must be remembered that periodontal diseases and most dental procedures may lead to gingival
bleeding. The mouth must, therefore, be regarded as a potentially
infectious site, and care must be taken to maintain proper infection
control procedures during dental radiography:

1.   It is recommended that all staff should wear gloves whenever
     intra-oral tissues are touched or manipulated, and that intra-oral

X-ray films should be wiped free of visible contamination when removed from the mouth.

2. Where a patient is identified as posing a particularly high risk of transmitting disease, then it may be advisable to use intra-oral films prewrapped in a plastic seal. The gloved operator can then carefully release the film from its wrapping, without contaminating the outer surface of the film envelope, and pass it for processing in the normal way. Caution is required, since unwrapping films for processing, wearing damp rubber gloves, may degrade the potential image with an overlying print.

3. If the film holders or other instruments are contaminated with blood or saliva, they should be washed free from visible contamination and sterilized immediately, in an autoclave or hot air oven, in the usual way. Modern plastic will survive sterilization in desk top sterilizers, as opposed to hot air sterilizers.

4. Any part of the dental chair or radiographic equipment which may have become contaminated with blood or saliva should be swabbed with a 1 per cent solution of domestic bleach (providing 1000 p/p/m available chlorine) and wiped dry. In the event of a larger spillage of blood, vomit, or other substance, the affected area should be treated with a 10 per cent solution of bleach, swabbed clean, and washed with a 1 per cent solution, before careful drying.

ACKNOWLEDGEMENT

With thanks to Dr Anita Sengupta for her dental anatomy contribution with illustrations.

FURTHER READING AND REFERENCES

Waite, E. (1996). *Essentials of dental radiography and radiology* (2nd edn). Churchill Livingstone.

Brocklebank, L. (1997). *Dental radiology: understanding the X-ray image*. Oxford University Press, Oxford.

Rinn Corporation. (1989). *Intra-oral radiography with Rinn XCP/BIA instruments*. Rinn Corporation, Illinois.

NRPB. (1994). *Guidelines on radiology standards for primary dental care.*

7 Digital dental radiology: radiovisiography

7.1 INTRODUCTION

Today, computer technology has become commonplace in our lives, with the personal computer an essential instrument in general medical practice, and many dental practices.

Computer technology offers a space-saving way to store patients' notes and communication within the National Health Service. In the field of medical radiology, it has been used for over 20 years — computerized tomography has become an essential diagnostic tool, together with magnetic resonance imaging and digital fluoroscopy (see Chapters 13 and 14). Digital fluoroscopy is often used by medical imaging departments when sialography is undertaken (the salivary gland is injected with contrast, under direct visualization).

However, it is only recently that digital imaging has become readily available to the general dental practitioner. Images in digital form can be readily manipulated, stored, and retrieved on computer. Furthermore, technology makes the transmission of images (teleradiology) practicable. The general principles of digital imaging are:

1. The chemically produced radiograph is represented by data that is acquired in a parallel and continuous fashion known as analogue.

2. Computers use binary (0 or 1) language, where information is usually handled in 8-character 'words' called bytes.

3. If each character can be either 0 or 1, this results in 2^8 possible combinations ('words'), that is, 256 'words'. Thus, dental digital images are limited to 256 shades of grey.

4. Digital images are made up of pixels (picture elements), each allocated a shade of grey.

5. The spatial resolution of a digital system is heavily dependent upon the number of pixels available per millimetre of image.

6. It is this factor which often differentiates apparatus on the market — as well as the ease of use and, of course, cost.

Direct digital dental radiology is now possible with two methods — one uses charge–coupled devices (CCD), and the other, photostimulable phosphor imaging plates. Both methods can be used in the dental surgery with conventional personal computers (PCs).

7.2   THE CCD SYSTEM

A number of manufacturers produce equipment using the CCD system:

- Radio Visiography, 'RVG' (by Trophy)
- Sens-a-Ray (by Regam)
- Visualix (by Gendex)
- Flash-Dent (by Villa)
- Sidexis (by Siemens)
- CDR (by Schick)

These systems all use an intra-oral sensor connected directly, by cable, to the computer. The sensor contains (depending on the manufacturer) one of the following:

(1) a combination of a rare earth intensifying screen as the primary receptor, fibre-optical coupling to transmit the fluorescence, and a conventional light-sensitive CCD to collect it (RVG);

(2) a 'hardened' X-ray-sensitive CCD as the primary receptor (Sens-a-Ray, Sidexis, CDR);

(3) the same as (1) but with a system of lenses in place of the fibre optics (Flash-Dent);

(4) a combination of an intensifying screen and hardened CCD (Visualix).

The analogue output from the CCD is converted to a digital format which is displayed on a monitor immediately. Hard copies can be provided with a digital or laser printer (Figs 7.1 and 7.2).

Advantages

(1) Low radiation dose (about half that of E-speed film);

(2) instant image;

(3) image manipulation facilities.

Disadvantages

(1) Small receptor size of most systems (apart from the CDR) makes only single-tooth imaging, possible (although this, in turn, is useful for endodontics);

(2) bulky sensor with cable;

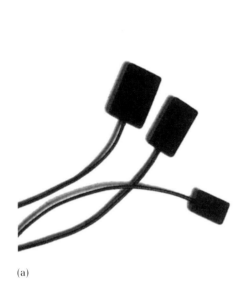

(a)

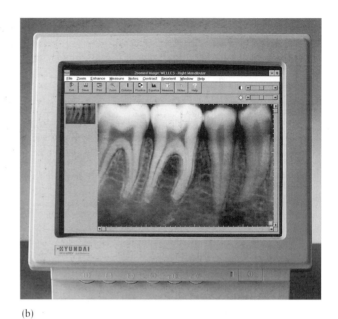

(b)

Fig. 7.1   CCD apparatus: (a) Schick
sensor; (b) Schick CDR; (c) Siemens
sidexis.

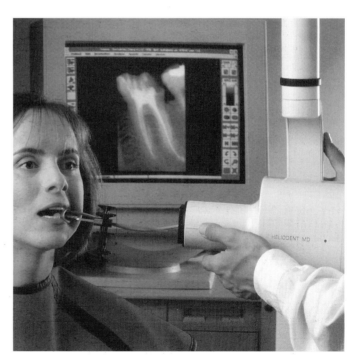

(c)

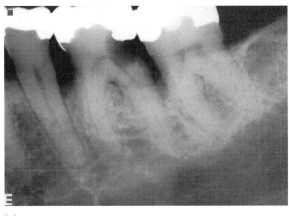

(a)

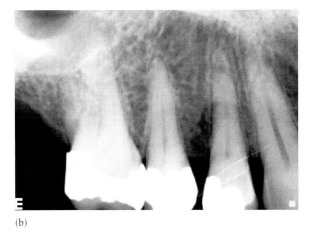

(b)

Fig. 7.2 Two sensor images: (a) lower molar region, demonstrating recurrence of caries in the ⌐6 and (b) an infra-bony defect is demonstrated distal to the ⌐4⌐.

(3) relative short life span of CCD (deterioration by X-ray bombardment);

(4) narrow exposure latitude ('burn out' of structures when sensor over-exposed);

(5) cost;

(6) storage of images can be a problem because of the need for special archiving equipment (optical disk, CD, large memory hard disk).

CCD systems for panoramic radiology are now available (Siemens, Planmeca) which use a linear CCD array corresponding in shape to the slit-collimated beam (see Chapter 10) (Fig. 7.3).

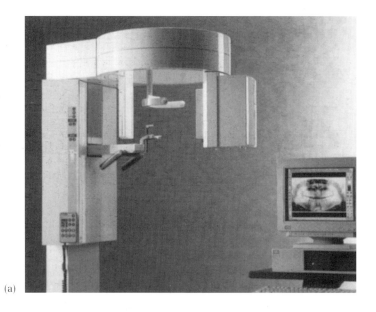

(a)

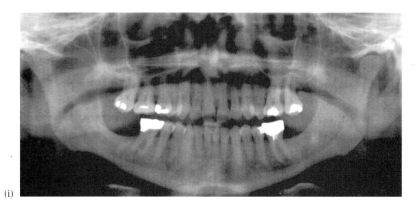

(i)

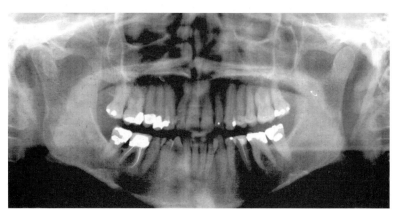

(ii)

Fig. 7.3   (a) Siemens Orthophos DS;
(b) examples of images.   (b)

7.3   PHOSPHOR IMAGING SYSTEM

At the present time, there is only one phosphor imaging system (Soredex-Digora) on the market. Whilst only recently introduced into the dental radiology field, it has been increasingly used in general radiology departments and in dental schools, where it has the great advantage that the computer processor and VDU can be remote from the X-ray apparatus and, therefore, service more than one apparatus. This would also be an advantage in multi-surgery practices (Fig. 7.4).

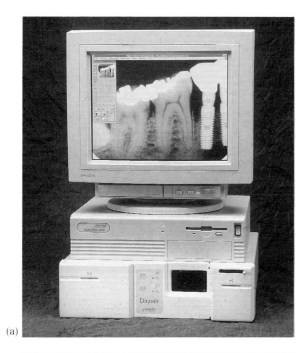

(a)

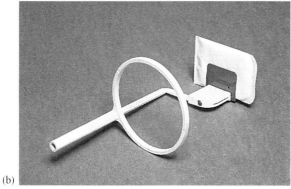

(b)

Fig. 7.4   (a) Soredex Digora; (b) film holders for imaging plates.

Key points

1. Chemical receptor —
   analogue image
2. Computer receptor —
   binary image

Digital dental systems
1. Charge-coupled devices
   (CCD) — use a sensor,
   connected by cable to the
   computer, which converts
   analogue image — to
   binary image, on screen,
   immediately on reception.
2. Phosphor imaging —
   imaging plate receives
   analogue image, converted
   to binary by 'processor', in
   30 seconds.
3. Advantages
   — low radiation dose
   — instant image
   — image manipulation
     facility
4. Disadvantages
   — hard receptor
   — narrow exposure
     latitude
   — cost
5. Fraudulent image potential

The photostimulable phosphor plates or sensors are the primary image receptor. These are coated with a layer containing europium-activated barium fluorohalide. When exposed to X-rays, some of the energy in the beam is stored by the phosphor. This 'latent image' of stored energy can then be released by subsequent scanning (inside a processing unit) by a laser beam of appropriate wavelength. The luminescence is magnified and detected by a photomultiplier tube and CCD, and displayed on a PC monitor. The sensors are available in two sizes and are reusable.

7.3.1   Practical instructions for 'processing'

1. Take an imaging plate and place it in one of the special plastic packages, ensuring that the seam on the package is facing the black surface of the plate.

2. Place the unsealed end of the package into the slot, on the left-hand side of the Digora, and press the button marked with the envelope icon — a green light flashes until it is sealed. Remove and use.

3. Expose the plate in the usual way, remembering that the same intra-oral techniques apply as with photographic-style radiographic film. The sensitive, white side is towards the tooth and X-ray beam. Imaging plate holders should be used with cotton wool rolls, if possible, as they are very hard and cannot be moulded.

4. Process the imaging plate with the Digora software programme on the computer:
   (a) The image can be assigned to a new patient card, or it can be added to an existing document;
   (b) The sealed envelope on the sensor is cut open, using the dedicated device, and inserted, without delay, into the scanner — white side facing left and the long axis vertical. Press the appropriate button according to the size of the imaging plate.

5. The image can be enhanced, if necessary, using the tools menu. For example, to demonstrate the root canal more clearly, increase the contrast.

6. Remove the imaging plate and replace for future use. Care must be taken with the imaging plate — though difficult, it is still possible to bend it, degrading any future use (Figs 7.5 and 7.6).

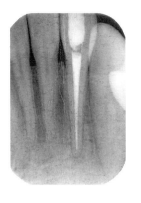

Fig. 7.5   (d) image of root-filled lower incisor (note the appearance of cracks running down the centre of the image, caused by bending of the imaging plate);

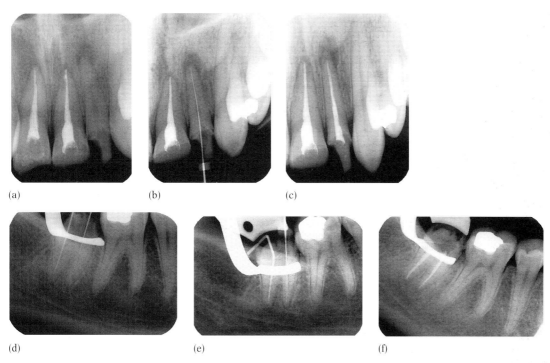

Fig. 7.6   Images taken with Digora direct digital system: (a) preoperative image of upper left lateral incisor, showing a periapical radiolucency; (b) image taken with file *in situ* for working length assessment; (c) image showing completed root filling (note the apparent increase in the vertical dimension of the periapical radiolucency — probably due to incorrect plate positioning, causing elongation rather than a true increase in size); (d) Image of lower right second molar, taken with endodontic files *in situ* for working length determination; (e) image taken with the master gutta percha cones *in situ*, prior to obturation; (f) image showing completed root canal filling.

Again, as with the CCD system, a hard copy can be obtained if necessary.

Advantages

(1) Low radiation dose (as low as 10 per cent of E-speed film);
(2) almost instant images (in approximately 20 seconds);
(3) very wide exposure latitude (it is almost impossible to 'burn out' information);
(4) same size receptors as film (therefore can be used for bitewings, and so on);
(5) X-ray source can be remote from PC;
(6) image manipulation facilities.

Disadvantages

(1) Cost;

(2) storage of images (same problem as CCD systems);

(3) slight inconvenience of protective bags.

7.4   THE FUTURE OF DENTAL DIGITAL IMAGING

7.4.1   Digital subtraction radiology

By digitally subtracting two images, taken using identical geometry but on different occasions, it is possible to produce an other image representing only the difference between the two. Using subtraction, it could be possible to monitor such things as caries progression, periodontal bone loss, and bone healing. This facility of subtraction is not (at the time of writing) available on any dental systems, and is principally a research tool. However, it is possible that the facility may be included on future versions of software.

In the medical sphere, digital fluoroscopy extends the subtraction principle with a facility to enhance the contrast medium (see Chapter 13). This has particular significance for dentists in sialography.

It must be understood that the success of subtraction is currently dependent upon a perfectly reproducible radiographic technique, if misinterpretations are not to be introduced. Hopefully, in the future, with more advances in technology, the general dental practitioner will have the advantage that, as the operator remains the same, the results will be comparable when monitoring a patient.

7.4.2   Computed image interpretation

Systems have been described which can identify and 'diagnose' caries and periapical lesions. However, such research is in its infancy. Very soon, computers in the dental surgery will include every aspect of management, accounting, patient records, as intra-oral video camera, as well as X-ray imaging and diagnosis.

7.5   FRAUDULENT IMAGE MANIPULATION

Legislation concerning computers is currently unclear. It is a relatively simple matter to use readily available computer software to 'alter' digital dental images. It remains to be seen whether this potential problem will result in safeguards being incorporated into digital systems, to ensure that the original image, can never be lost. The general dental practitioner would, in any case, be wise to keep the original image — in some countries within the EC, this is obligatory — as a check to prevent fraudulent alteration of images (Fig. 7.7).

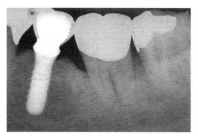

(a)

REFERENCES AND FURTHER READING

Horner, K. *et al.* (1996). Potential medico-legal implications of computed radiography. *British Dental Journal*, **180**, **No. 7**, 271–3.

Waite, E. (1996). *Essentials of dental radiography and radiology* (2nd edn). Churchill Livingstone.

Visser, H. and Kruger, W. (1997). Can dentists recognise manipulated digital radiographs? *Journal of the International Association of Dentomaxillofacial Radiology*, **26**, No.1, 67–9.

Price, C. and Ergul, N.A. (1997). Comparison of film based and a direct digital dental radiographic system using a proximal caries model. *Journal of the International Association of Dentomaxillofacial Radiology*, **26**, No.1, 45–52.

White, S.C. and Yvon, D.C. (1997). Comparative performance of digital and conventional images for detecting proximal caries. *Journal of the International Association of Dentomaxillofacial Radiology*, **26**, No.1, 32–44.

Wenzel, A. and Grondahl H.G. (1995). Direct digital radiography in the dental office. *International Dental Journal*, **45**, 27–34.

Curry, T.S., Dowdry, J.E., and Murray, R.C. (1990). *Chrisrensen's Physics of Diagnostic Radiology*, fourth edition. Lea & Febiger, Philadelphia.

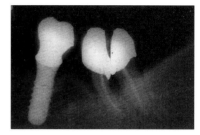

(b)

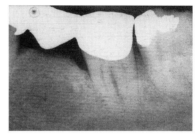

(c)

Fig. 7.7 An example of a manipulated radiograph: (a) was composed from the radiographs of two patients, (b) and (c). (Reproduced from *Journal of the International Association of entomaxillofacial Radiology*, **26**, 67–9. Reproduced with kind permission of H. Visser and W. Kruge.)

8 Occlusal radiography

8.1 INTRODUCTION

Occlusal radiography includes all techniques employed when films are positioned in the occlusal plane. These projections may be undertaken with the patient in the vertical or in the working position. It may be more comfortable for the patient to begin in the working position, especially for radiographs of the mandible, as long as some support is placed under the neck.

The important factor is the position of the occlusal plane and its relationship to the X-ray beam. Placing the patient in the midline will not be difficult in either the vertical or working position. Lateral views will require more judgement — in either position, the head has to be adjusted to make the required angulation with the X-ray beam (Fig. 8.1).

Usually, a 5.7 × 7.6 cm film is used, though periapical films may be sufficient in paedodontics. Where no occlusal films are available, two adjacent periapicals would be a reasonable substitute. A larger area is demonstrated in occlusal radiography, and the film is placed between the occlusal surfaces of the teeth.

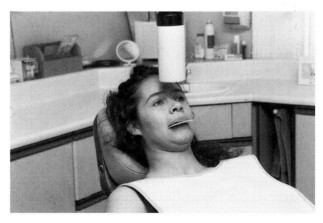

Fig. 8.1 The patient in the working position for a central upper occlusal. The X-ray beam is vertical, so the occlusal plane is raised 20° from the horizontal to ensure that the beam and the film will have the correct angulation to each other — 70°.

Occlusal radiography can be separated into two groups:

1. *True occlusal*
This occlusal projection will demonstrate the shape of the dental arch, the palate and the floor of the mouth, the buccal and lingual plates, and part of the antra. It will make it possible:

(a) to determine the true position and direction of normal or displaced teeth and tooth fragments;
(b) to assess the extent to which lesions are affecting the structure around a tooth, and to delineate cyst formations and bone expansion — in other words, to establish the degree of neoplastic invasion;
(c) to study bone formation on the buccal and lingual surfaces of the mandible and maxilla, and, Consequently, to help determine the true relationship of the fragments of a fracture;
(d) to demonstrate calculi in the submandibular gland and duct.

Ideally, the X-ray beam should be directed perpendicular to the film, from above or below. When the X-ray beam is directed down the long axis of the tooth or teeth to be examined, or perpendicular to the area of the mandible or maxilla to be demonstrated, it can be used in combination with the periapical projection or relevant extra-oral views (see Chapter 9).

2. *Oblique or topographical occlusal* Films placed between occlusal surfaces of the teeth can be an extension of the bisecting angle periapical technique.

In paedodontics, this projection is often easier to achieve as it covers a larger area, it will demonstrate unerupted teeth for the orthodontist. In cases of trauma — where the usual periapical films are impossible to use — and in very narrow arches, it can be invaluable.

Oblique occlusals demonstrate:

- the area of the mandible and maxilla beyond the apex
- fractures
- the full extent of a cyst
- unerupted teeth and supernumaries
- if not too high, a root in the antrum.

8.2   PLACEMENT OF FILM IN MOUTH

In order to avoid discomfort to the patient, the film should be inserted with care into the mouth Gently curve the film so that it goes into the

Key points

1. True occlusal projections demonstrate the dental arches at right angles to the occlusal plane
2. Oblique occlusal projections demonstrate larger areas of the maxilla and mandible than can be seen on periapical film

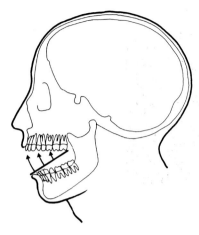

Fig. 8.2   Diagram to show how to insert the occlusal film into the mouth.

oral cavity without unnecessary stretching of the corners of the mouth. It is helpful to place only the posterior edge of the film as far back as necessary, at an angle to the occlusal plane, and then raise or lower the film into position. When this method is used, the patient will be less likely to gag than when the whole film is just pushed back as far as possible (Fig. 8.2).

Edentulous patients should be allowed to retain the opposite denture from the jaw under investigation, to prevent the film from slipping. Placing one or two cotton wool rolls between the alveolar process and the film will make an angle adjustment for the absence of crowns unnecessary. In cases where the absence of teeth causes the film to lie unevenly, cotton wool rolls should be used to balance the bite.

The film should be held in position by the firm, but not overly so, bite of the patient. Over-vigorous clenching of the teeth will mark the film and spoil the diagnostic value of the radiograph.

8.3   LOWER JAW PROJECTIONS

Central true occlusal view of the mandible and floor of mouth

The patient sits or reclines in the dental chair, with the occlusal plane as near vertical as possible. It is sometimes easier for elderly patients to stand with support, and for the X-ray beam to be directed from below. Place the film transversely in the mouth.

- *Centring point*: 3 cm below the symphysis menti in the midline.
- *Direction of X-ray beam*: 90° to the occlusal plane and the film.
- *Anode–film distance*: 30–40 cm

In this case, the object is very wide, and to obtain a true occlusal projection of as much of it as possible, the anode–film distance should be at least 30 cm. Remember, the longer the anode–film distance, the more parallel the X-ray beam. Nevertheless, care must be taken that the collimating device enables the filed of irradiation to be precisely curtailed. The co-operation of the patient and the length of the exposure time must be taken into account, as this is an uncomfortable position to maintain (Fig. 8.3).

Anterior true lower occlusal view

For the incisor region, the film should be placed in the occlusal plane, but the posterior edge should not be much further back than the pre-

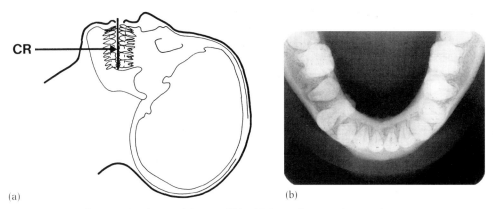

(a) (b)

Fig. 8.3 Central true occlusal view of the mandible: (a) direct the central ray in the median plane perpendicular to the occlusal plane, 3 cm below the symphysis menti; (b) this projection demonstrates a supplementary tooth in the right first premolar region, presenting lingually.

molars. This will allow enough film for the image, which may be projected labially.

- *Centring point*: the symphysis menti.
- *Direction of X-ray beam*: up the root canals of the incisors. (This will usually be 10–20° greater than the central view; 100–110° to the film.)
- *Anode–film distance*: 30 cm

(Fig. 8.4.) (See also Figs 9.9 and 9.18)

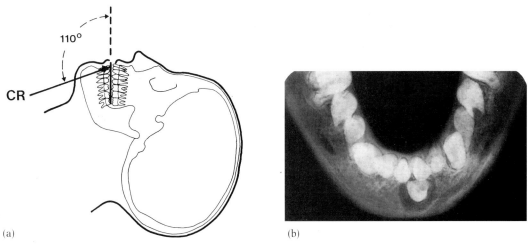

(a) (b)

Fig. 8.4 Lower arch anterior true occlusal: (a) direct the central ray up the root canals of the incisor teeth under the symphysis menti; (b) this projection demonstrates the unerupted incisor within the cyst, buccal to the erupted teeth. It also demonstrates an odontome relative to the uccal. (See Figs 9.9 and 9.18, for other views of the same patient.)

True lateral lower occlusal

The film is displaced to the side of the mandible under investigation, with the long axis parallel to the lie of the row of teeth.

- *Centring point*: 4 cm above the angle of the mandible.
- *Direction of X-ray beam*: 90° to the film, and parallel to the lateral surface of the mandible (that is, 10–15° to the median plane).
- *Anode–film distance*: 30 cm

(Fig. 8.5)

This technique can be extended to any section of the mandible if:

(1) the film is placed centrally behind the area under investigation;

(2) the X-ray beam centred over this is at 90° and follows the line of the mandible at that point.

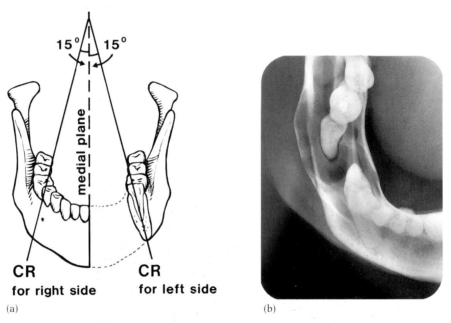

(a) (b)

Fig. 8.5 Lower lateral true occlusal: (a) direct the central ray 15° to the median plane, centring over the first molar parallel to the lateral surface of the mandible; (b) this projection demonstrates the lingual and buccal expansion of the cortical plates of the mandible. The cyst is pseudoloculated and involves submerged premolar teeth.

Lower occlusal for unerupted third molar and submandibular gland

When the angle of the mandible or unerupted third molar lying in the ascending ramus is to be demonstrated, the film should be placed as far back as in the mouth possible. The head should be tilted back to

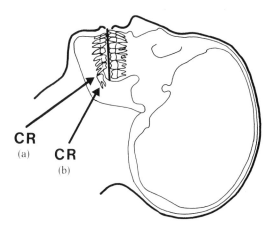

Fig. 8.6 Lower lateral oblique true occlusal for the unerupted third molar and for stones in the posterior portion of the submandibular duct: (a) central ray directed about 100° to the film, between the distal edge of the crown of the second molar and the unerupted third molar; (b) central beam directed 110° through the angle of the mandible, towards the occlusal plane parallel to the ascending ramus.

place the occlusal plane near the vertical, and then rotated away from the affected side. It is then possible to centre the X-ray beam over the angle of the mandible, directing the beam upwards by 20–25°, but still keeping to the line of the mandible.

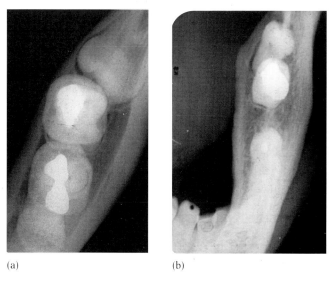

Fig. 8.7 (a) Lateral true occlusal, centred to show the horizontal third molar in its relationship to the second molar; (b) lower lateral oblique true occlusal demonstrating a horizontal third molar lying obliquely across the line of the arch.

- *Centring point*: the angle of the mandible or the submandibular gland.
- *Direction of X-ray beam*: 110–115° to the film and parallel to the ascending ramus.
- *Anode–film distance*: 30 cm

It is possible to use a periapical film for the impacting third molar. This is most useful when information as to the exact relationship between the second molar and the unerupted tooth is required. The central ray should then be directed parallel to the distal surface of the second molar. Less angulation to the film — 95–100° — is often required (Figs 8.6 and 8.7). This is a useful view when examining the salivary ducts and gland, see Fig. 13.1a, 13.4b.

Lower midline oblique occlusal

It is sometimes necessary to obtain a view of the lower anterior region of the mandible, to demonstrate the full depth from the crowns of the incisors to the lower border. This same view can be used for small children who will not co-operate with a periapical film, or in the case of a very narrow arch, where it is impossible to avoid excessive curvature of the film using the normal periapical technique.

The patient's head should be supported comfortably, with the film placed in the occlusal plane back to the premolar region.

- *Centring point*: the symphysis menti.
- *Direction of X-ray beam*: in the midline, 45° to the plane of the film.
- *Anode–film distance*: 20 cm

(Figs 8.8 and 8.9)

This technique can be extended to other areas of the mandible, the same principles applying:

1. The object is in the centre of the film.
2. The X-ray beam is directed at right angles to a tangent, at the area under investigation.
3. The X-ray beam is 35–45° to the film.

(Fig. 8.10)

8.4   UPPER JAW PROJECTIONS

In the maxilla, the difference in the angulation of the incisor teeth to the occlusal plane, compared to the relationship of the molar teeth to this plane, make a true occlusal projection of this arch particularly

---

Key points

Mandible
1. Central true occlusal — X-ray-beam 90° to film in midline
2. Anterior true occlusal — X-ray-beam 115° upwards through lower incisors
3. Lateral true occlusal — X-ray-beam 90° to film over to one side of arch, towards median plane
4. Posterior lateral occlusal — X-ray-beam centred over the angle of the mandible for lower 3rd molar upwards 20–25° in line with the mandible
5. Lower midline occlusal — X-ray-beam 35–45° to the film can be applied to other areas of mandible

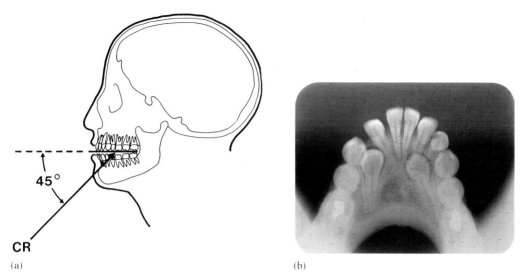

(a)   (b)

Fig. 8.8 Anterior middle oblique lower occlusal: (a) direct central ray in the mid line at 45° to the occlusal plane; (b) this view was taken to demonstrate unerupted canines in a patient with a narrow and crowded arch.

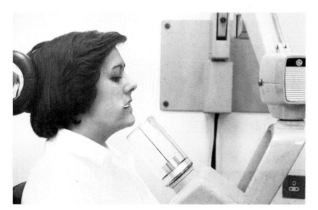

Fig. 8.9 Patient sitting vertically with central ray 45° to the occlusal plane.

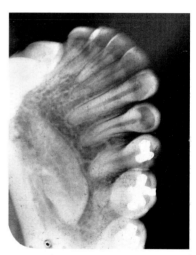

Fig. 8.10 Oblique lower occlusal in the left premolar showing an unerupted canine from the other side of the mandible.

difficult. The problem is compounded by the superimposition of the frontal bone. Because of the anatomical variation in the shape of this bone, when the X-ray beam is directed at right angles to the true occlusal plane, the relationship of the frontal bone with the maxilla will also be variable. In some cases, it will completely superimpose the maxilla and, in others hardly at all. This causes problems with exposure factors due to the extremes in density.

Where the frontal bone is superimposed, there is a lack of detail, and intensifying screens (see Chapter 2), will be necessary. These cut down the amount of radiation necessary and, consequently, reduce the fogging caused by the scattering rays.

In practice, a true, overall occlusal view of the maxilla is seldom attempted. When the exact position of unerupted anterior supernumaries or unerupted canines is to be demonstrated, in their relationship with the central incisors, a vertex occlusal is taken. For a general view demonstrating the presence of unerupted teeth, the pathological conditions of the maxilla, or fractures, a compromise view is taken — a 'central occlusal' of the maxilla.

Vertex occlusal for the incisor region

This view should be taken with the use of intensifying screens which are sized to fit the occlusal film (Fig. 8.11(a)).

For hygienic reasons, place the occlusal cassette in a small plastic bag. Support the patient's head and place the cassette into the mouth, asking the patient to hold it in position against the upper teeth (with both thumbs). The cassette must be held so that it is in contact only with the anterior teeth, see Fig. 8.11b.

This may be achieved with the X-ray beam vertical and the teeth brought into the line of the rays (Fig. 8.12). It may also be achieved by directing the X-ray beam from the vertex, forward along the line of the root canals (see Fig. 8.11 (b)).

- *Centring point*: midline over the central incisors.
- *Direction of X-ray beam*: parallel with the root canals of the central incisors.
- *Anode–film distance*: 45 cm

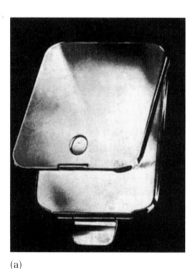

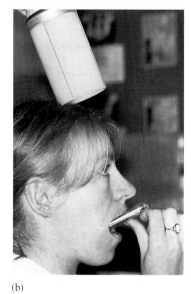

Fig. 8.11 (a) Occlusal cassette incorporating intensifying screens; (b) occlusal cassette being used for a vertex occlusal projection.

(a)

(b)

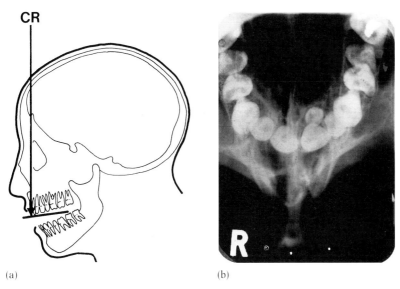

(a)   (b)

Fig. 8.12   Anterior vertex occlusal: (a) direct central ray down root canals of central incisors; (b) an unerupted supernumerary in the upper left incisor region.

Central vertex occlusal

This projection is seldom take — occasionally, for the exact position of unerupted upper premolars.

Place the occlusal cassette, in its protective bag, between the crowns of the teeth, taking care not to allow the patient to bite too hard on the metal casing, so distorting it. If lead rubber is used to prevent back scatter when the beam penetrates into the mouth, this also helps with the bite. The occlusal plane is in the horizontal.

• *Centring point and direction of X-ray beam*: centre over the frontal bone, about 20° to the vertical, to allow the central ray to pass down the root canals of the premolars.
• Anode–film distance: 45 cm
(Fig. 8.13)

Central upper occlusal

This is a modified technique to avoid superimposition of the frontal bone.

• *Centring point*: root of the nose (nasion).
• *Direction of X-ray beam*: 70–80° down the sagittal plane. The angle will depend upon the area of the maxilla to be investigated and the shape of the frontal bone.
• *Anode–film distance*: 30 cm
(Fig. 8.14)

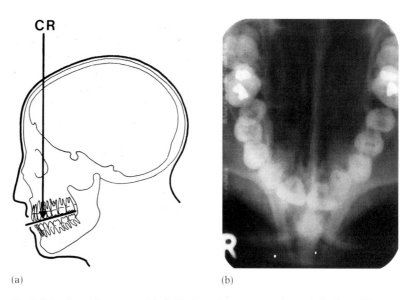

(a)　　　　　　　　　　(b)

Fig. 8.13   Central vertex occlusal: (a) direct beam to pass through the frontal bone, through the premolar region, on to the cassette; (b) this projection demonstrates a patalally placed premolar. The anterior teeth are seen in an oblique projection.

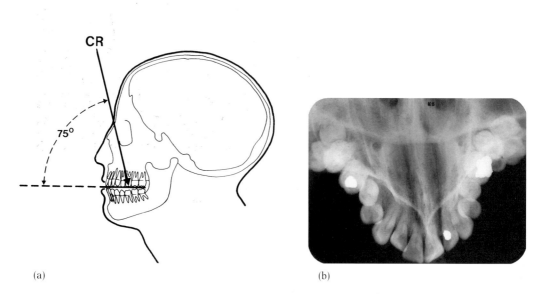

(a)　　　　　　　　　　(b)

Fig. 8.14   Central upper occlusal: (a) direct central ray at 75° to the occlusal plane, through the nasion; (b) with the film placed transversely, this projection shows the relative position of unerupted molars and supernumerary teeth to the erupted teeth in the molar region.

It is only necessary to give sufficient angle to throw the frontal bone clear of the area under examination. If only one side is required, place the film to the affected side. If both molar regions are required, place the film in the mouth with the long axis at right angles to the median plane. If necessary, the incisors may be excluded. This position of the film may be uncomfortable for the patient, so speed is essential — centre the X-ray tube before inserting the film into the mouth.

Upper midline oblique-anterior occlusal view

This projection will demonstrate anterior teeth and the presence of supernumaries, and is comparable to that described earlier under 'lower anterior oblique occlusal'. It is also very useful for young children when a periapical film may be placed horizontally between anterior teeth, see Fig. 5.22 — otherwise use an occlusal film inserted [n the long axis] enough to include the incisor region.

- *Centering point*: bridge of nose
- *Direction of X-ray beam*: 60–65° down the sagittal plane.
- *Anode–film distance*: 30 cm

(Fig. 8.15)

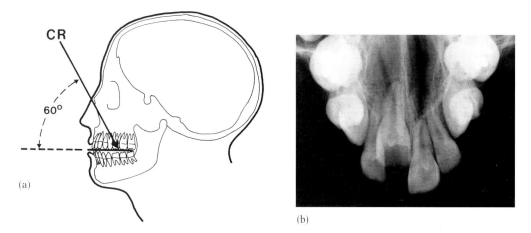

(a)

(b)

Fig. 8.15　Upper midline oblique occlusal: (a) direct the central ray at 60° to the occlusal plane, over the bridge of the nose; (b) this view demonstrates an unerupted central incisor.

Upper oblique occlusal view

This view:

(1) demonstrates fractures;

(2) highlights many pathological conditions involving large areas of the maxilla;

Key points

Maxilla
1. Frontal bone can be superimposed
2. Vertex occlusal — X-ray beam 90° to film
3. Central occlusal — 70° to film in the median plane; centre over nasion
4. Lateral oblique occlusal — 60° through floor of orbit

(3) provides an auxiliary view for palatal roots of the molar teeth, when the malar bone obscures the roots in the periapical view;

(4) is one of the views taken to demonstrate a root in the antrum.

Place the film in the mouth longitudinally. The film should project laterally, just beyond the cusps of the teeth under investigation.

- *Centring point*: between the canine and the first molar region, depending upon the area required, at the same level as the nasion.
- *Direction of X-ray beam*: 60–65° down through the floor of orbit.
- *Anode–film distance*: 30 cm

Do not centre the beam posterior to the outer canthus of the eye, as this will cause the zygomatic bone and arch to be superimposed over the maxilla. It is very important that the lateral direction of the X-ray beam is correct. Direct the beam to the curve of the maxilla, as for periapical views, between the canine and premolar regions (Fig. 8.16).

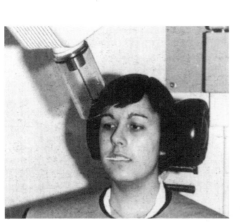

(a)

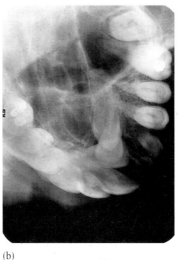

(b)

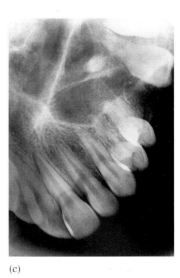

(c)

Fig. 8.16 (a) Patient positioned for upper lateral oblique occlusal; (b) this view taken to demonstrate the canine region, showing a cyst related to the crown and dilacerated central incisor; (c) this projection confirms the presence of a root in the maxillary antrum.

REFERENCES AND FURTHER READING

Waites, E. (1996). *Essentials of dental radiography and radiology* (2nd ed). Churchill Livingstone, London.

Brocklebank, L. (1997). *Dental Radiology: understanding the image.* Oxford University Press, Oxford.

Taj, C. C., Miller, P. A., Packota, G. V., Wood, R. E. (1994). *The occlusal radiograph revisited Oral-Health*, **84**(11), 47–80.

9　Extra-oral radiography: I

In all these radiographic techniques, the film is placed outside the oral cavity, either against the side of the face to be radiographed or nearby, and the X-ray beam is directed towards it. The techniques can be divided into the following categories:

- those undertaken in general dental practice
- those undertaken in maxillo facial imaging departments. Within this category the advanced imaging techniques include computerized tomography, magnetic resonance imaging and ultrasound — all considered in later chapters.

9.1　TECHNIQUES FOR GENERAL DENTAL PRACTICE

1. *Oblique lateral technique*
These views demonstrate:

(a) larger areas of the mandible — from the condyle and coronoid, to the symphysis menti, and the maxilla — than can be shown with the intra-oral films;
(b) fractures of the mandible, usually in conjunction with occlusal views to get two views at right angles to each other;
(c) unerupted teeth lying below the apexes or third molars impacting into the ascending ramus;
(d) the full extent of pathological conditions.

In the case of trismus, it is often the only technique possible for dental practitioners, if they do not have panoramic apparatus.

2. *Auxiliary views taken with a dental X-ray unit without a grid.*
This technique may be used to demonstrate:

(a) foreign bodies in soft tissue;
(b) a true lateral of the nasal bones, to establish the presence of a fracture;

(c) true lateral and tangential views of the maxilla or mandible, demonstrating buccally placed teeth, possibly associated with pathology.

3. Dental panoramic tomography

This is a specialized form of sectional tomography, whereby tomograms are made of curved layers. It presents a panoramic view of the facial bones, with 'unfolding' of the maxilla and mandible (see Chapter 11). A large number of dentists now include this apparatus within their general practice as a valuable tool in diagnosis.

4. Cephalometry

This technique demonstrates views of the facial bones, using a stable head immobilizer (a craniostat) in order to obtain the comparable projections which are often necessary when assessing patients before and during orthodontic treatment. Many manufactures market apparatus for general practice which allow the same X-ray tube to be utilized for either the panoramic or the cephalometric mode, for example, the Siemens Orthophos Plus (see Fig. 11.13, p. 183).

This chapter covers radiographic techniques in the first two categories. Radiography of the facial bones including cephalometry and dental panoramic tomography are dealt with in Chapters 10 and 11.

9.2   OBLIQUE LATERAL RADIOGRAPHY

Oblique lateral radiography presents certain problems because of the anatomical structure of the mandible and maxilla. There is, a therefore a tendency to regard this method of examination as difficult to explain and even more difficult to execute. The basic problem is one of superimposition — of the structures on the opposite side of the face, the cervical spine, and, for the mandible, of the hyoid bone — and in solving this problem, not to produce a radiograph which is elongated and distorted.

If the mandible is considered anatomically, it is seen to be horseshoe shaped. As with the intra-oral techniques, it is necessary to divide it into separate segments:

- condyle and ascending ramus
- molar
- premolar
- canine and incisor regions.

The head must, therefore, be rotated so that the area under examination is parallel to the film (Fig. 9.1).

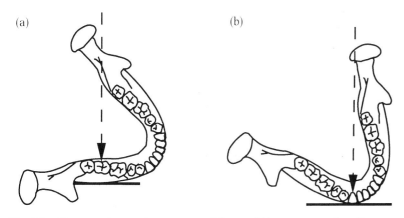

Fig. 9.1   Diagrams showing how rotation of the mandible is necessary for oblique lateral radiographs of (a) the molar; (b) the canine regions.

Superimposition of spine
The more mesial the region to be radiographed, the greater must be the rotation. In order to limit the superimposition of the spinal shadow, the mandible must be extended away from the spine. It is always possible to prevent the superimposition of the spine over the particular segment under examination. This uplifting of the chin will also even out the soft tissue, which might otherwise cause an unnecessarily dense area adjacent to the spine.

Superimposition of the opposite side of the face
This can be overcome by the combination of an angle between the sagittal plane and the film, and the angulation of the X-ray beam.

- Position the head to achieve an angle of 10° between the sagittal plane and the film;
- Position the X-ray beam at 10° towards the vertex.
- The addition of the 10° angle of the sagittal plane to the film and the X-ray beam 10° angulation, will make an effective separation of 20°.
- If the angle of the sagittal plane or the film is increased on its own, the angulation necessary to separate one side from the other will result in elongation of the object.

The centring point remains more or less the same whichever segment is being radiographed, as the opposite angle will rotate with the head.

The oblique lateral technique uses these basic principles, and no additional equipment is required. It can be adapted for different situations

— so long as the relative positioning of the head and X-ray beam is understood — and undertaken:

(1) with the patient seated and leaning over a horizontal surface — easiest way to assess; and position the head;

(2) with the patient horizontal — easy to immobilize;

(3) with the patient vertical.

Position 1

The patient is seated upright and sideways in a chair or stool, by the side of a horizontal surface. Either the stool or the table must be adjustable to adapt to the height of the patient. The patient's head is lowered, vertex downwards, on to the film, so that the sagittal plane makes the angle of 10° with the horizontal. (In this way, the side of the mandible under examination will be parallel to the film, and the opposite side angled away in an upward plane.) (Fig. 9.2) Angle the X-ray beam at 10° and centre over the opposite angle of the mandible.

Position 2

With the patient in the working position, he or she can be rotated to the side under examination. The dental chair may be lowered so that

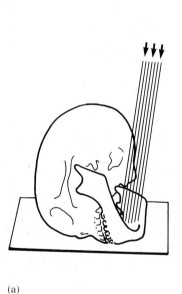

(a)

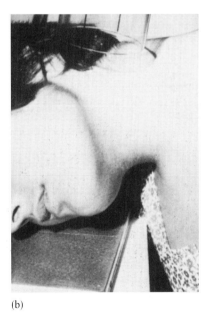

(b)

Fig. 9.2   (a) Diagram showing position for an oblique lateral radiograph of the mandible in the molar region. The side of the mandible to be X-rayed is parallel to the film and the opposite site is angled away in an upward plane. (b) Oblique lateral radiograph with the patient seated. The head is in the horizontal plane and the central ray is directed over the opposite angle of the jaw at 10° towards the vertex.

the head can decline at 10°. The cassettte is placed on the head-rest and the patient's head positioned on to it, still keeping the sagittal plane parallel to the film. Failing this, lower the sagittal plane to make the 10° angle with the film and the consequent separation of one side of the mandible from the other, as in the previous instance. Alternately, it may be helpful to use a 10° foam wedge-shaped pad (Fig. 9.3).

The head is now rotated so that the segment to be examined is exactly parallel to the film.

Tilt the head back on the spine, to extend the mandible away from it.

Angle the X-ray beam at 10° and centre over the opposite angle of the mandible.

Position 3
With the patient seated vertically in the dental chair, holding the film, the sagittal plane of the head is inclined 10° towards the film, and the X-ray beam angled upwards (Fig. 9.4).

If the mandible and the maxilla are to be demonstrated together, whichever position of the head is used, this combined angulation of the saaggital plane to the film at 10° X-ray beam can be taken as the

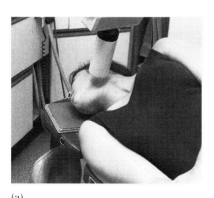
(a)

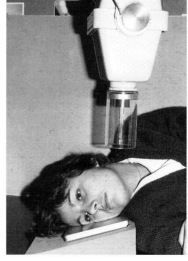
(b)

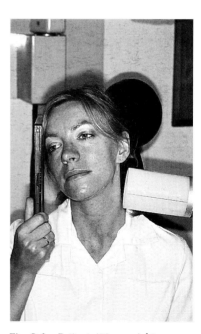

Fig. 9.3 (a) Patient lying on the dental chair, moving over from the working position so that the molar region is parallel to the cassette. (b) Patient lying horizontally, with the head positioned for the oblique lateral technique. An plastic foam wedge is sometimes useful to achieve the necessary separation of one mandible from the other.

Fig. 9.4 Patient sitting upright, holding film vertical. The sagittal plane is angled 10° towards the film. The central ray is directed 10° towards the vertical.

constant separation of one side of the mandible from the other. If it is impossible to place the vertex of the patient's head downwards, to make the full 10° to the table, or vertically towards the film, then the angle of the X-ray beam must be increased — despite the resultant elongation. In most cases, when both the mandible and the maxilla are needed together to demonstrate unerupted teeth, the patient is young and co-operative.

- For the mandible only, the sagittal plane angle is not so necessary and, in fact, should not be too great, as the hyoid bone may become superimposed over the object.
- When the maxilla, alone, is to be demonstrated, the centring points should be 2 cm behind and 2 cm above the opposite angle of the mandible, which will in itself help to clear the other mandible out of the way. A further rotation of 5° is also helpful.
- The important fact with this technique is to keep the angulation of the X-ray beam to a minimum to avoid elongation. The tilt of the sagittal plane will tend to cancel out the elongation effect of the X-ray beam as it foreshortens the object, whilst the addition of the two angles will give the required separation with minimum distortion.

Intensifying screens (see Ch. 2)

The oblique lateral technique requires the use of intensifying screens, which should be of as high definition as possible. The need for bone detail must be weighted against the level of radiation dosage. Remember, the faster the screens, the smaller the margin of error with exposure factors (see Chapter 2).

The anode–film distance (see Ch. 2)

If the required increase in area is to projected on to film, the anode–film distance must be at least 30 cm. The greater the anode–film distance the less the enlargement of the image. Ideally, with the appropriate equipment, an anode–film distance of 75–90 cm will give the best results, together with a small diaphragm and appropriate collimator device, to reduce the area irradiated to a minimum.

The head should be immobilized with the aid of sandbags or a headband, and a foam wedge is useful as a chin rest.

Angle boards

An angle board can be used to support the film either in the vertical or the horizontal. It is particularly useful in the vertical position, helping to achieve the required separation of one side of the mandible from the other. If the two mandibular angles are level, even an angle board will not separate them.

Remember that the sagittal plane must be parallel to the film, and care must be taken when rotating the face towards the film not to lose this relationship. If the X-ray tube can be extended far enough, the patient may support the film against a wall and the sagittal plane can then be angled towards it, achieving the same relationship as when the film is horizontal. Exactly the same technique can be used in hospital with a cassette holder (see Fig. 9.4). Elderly and ill patients find the erect position more comfortable.

This method generally inclines the film at 10–20°, and so the angle on the X-ray beam may be lowered accordingly (Fig. 9.5).

To summarize this technique in a way that is easy to remember, let us take the position most frequently required — the molar region — with the head in the horizontal position, lowered, vertex downwards.

When the patient is horizontal, starting from the working position, it is relatively simple for him or her to move over on their side and achieve the position described below. When the patient is sitting upright, then the instructions are adapted through 90°. So, for example, the sagittal plane is then inclined 10° to the vertical instead of the horizontal.

9.2.1 Mandible with maxilla

Molar region

- *Sagittal plane* 10° to the horizontal.
- *Rotation*: 10–15° from the true lateral.
- *Extension of the mandible*: 10° from the spine.
- *X-ray beam*: 10° towards the vertex.
- *Centring point*: opposite angle of the mandible.

(Fig. 9.6)

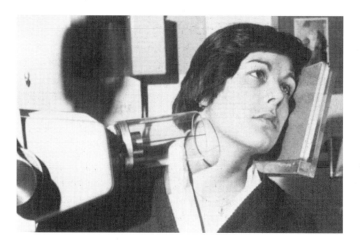

> **Key points**
>
> *Extra-oral oblique-lateral projections of the mandible and maxilla*
>
> Divided into 4 regions:
> — condyle and ascending ramus
> — molar
> — premolar
> — canine and incisor
>
> *Problems*
>
> Superimposition of the spine:
> — rotate head towards film
> — raise chin
>
> Superimposition of opposite jaws:
> — angle sagittal plane to film
> — angle X-ray-beam to vertex

> **Key points**
>
> *Four angles of 10°*
> 1. Sagittal plane, towards the film
> 2. Rotation from the lateral, towards the film
> 3. Extension of the mandible, from the spine
> 4. X-ray beam, angle, centred from the spine

Fig. 9.5 Patient sitting upright in the dental chair, with the sagittal plane inclined at 15° to the vertical and parallel to the angle board and the film. The central ray is directed at 5° to the vertex.

For other regions of the mandible and the maxilla, the important variable is the rotation of the head.

Ramus

- *Rotation*: the head is only slightly rotated towards the film, away from the true lateral.
- *Extension of the mandible*: as much as possible.
- Sagittal plane and a maximum combined separation is necessary of 20–25° X-ray beam

(Fig. 9.7)

Premolar region

- *Sagittal plane*: 10° to the horizontal.
- *Rotation*: the head is rotated until the region is parallel to the film.
- *Extension of the mandible*: as much as possible.
- *X-ray beam*: the angulation is increased 10–15° to the vertex. This will increase the separation of the mandible and demonstrate a wider area of the jaws. In children, when the molar and premolar regions are required on one film, to diagnose the presence of unerupted teeth the slight elongation will not detract from this.
- *Centring point*: opposite angle of the mandible.

(Fig. 9.8)

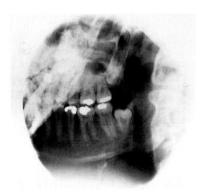

Fig. 9.6   Oblique lateral taken to demonstrate unerupted upper and lower third molars.

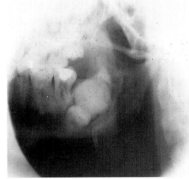

Fig. 9.7   Oblique lateral view of the ramus and molar region showing odontome associated with 8/ extending half-way up the ramus, almost to the level of the lingular.

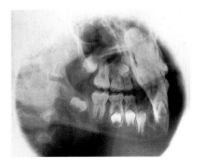

Fig. 9.8   Oblique lateral view of the premolar region in a 7-year-old child, demonstrating presence and position of unerupted teeth.

Canine and incisor region:

- *Sagittal plane*: 5° to the horizontal.
- *Rotation*: as far as possible, flattening the patient's nose. The amount of rotation will vary according to the shape of the jaws — the segment to be examined must be parallel to the film. As the head is rotated to the canine and incisor regions, the sagittal plane lessens. This is not important because the opposite side is being rotated away, but if no angulation of the sagittal plane is attempted, it is difficult to place the required area parallel to the film without some superimposition of the opposite side.
- *Extension of the mandible*: as much as possible.
- *X-ray beam*: 10° to the vertex.
- *Centring point*: 2 cm behind the opposite angle of the mandible. (Fig. 9.9)

9.2.2   The mandible

The radiographic technique remains the same for each area as just described, except for the angle of separation.

- The mandible alone does not require so much separation — either the sagittal plane or the X-ray beam angle may be reduced.
- The amount of separation will not be constant if the superimposition of the hyoid bone is to be avoided.
- As with so much else in this work, it will vary with the individual. In some patients, a 10° inclination to the vertex will throw the opposite mandible clear of the maxilla, and yet at the same

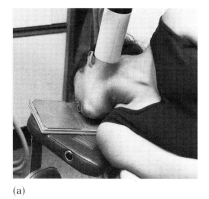
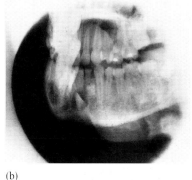

(a)   (b)

Fig. 9.9   (a) Patient in the working position of the dental chair, moving over so that the canine region is parallel to the film (b) oblique lateral rotated for the canine and incisor region. There is a retained B, the root of which is associated with an odontome. Just anterior to this is an uperupted tooth within a dentigerous cyst. (The same patient is demonstrated in Fig. 8.4, p. 137 and Fig. 9.18)

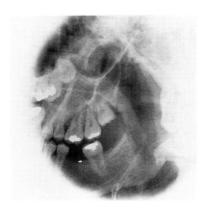

Fig. 9.10   Oblique lateral for maxillary molar teeth showing impacted third molar.

Key points

Variables

1. Mandible alone
   — not too much angle of separation
   — superimposition of hyoid

2. Maxilla alone
   — rotate 5° more towards film
   — centre behind and above opposite angle

---

time, the hyiod bone will still be below the lower border of the region to be examined. At the other extreme, it may be impossible to clear the opposite mandible from the crown, and the hyoid bone from the apex of a tooth in the mandible adjacent to the film.

9.2.3   The maxilla

- *Rotation*: 5° more towards the film than usual.
- *Centring point*: 2 cm behind and 2 cm above the opposite angle of the mandible.

(Fig. 9.10)

9.2.4   Bimolar radiography

This is, in fact, a misnomer, for it was a technique originally devised to demonstrate unerupted teeth in children requiring orthodontic treatment. Both sides of the face can be radiographed on one film — this is useful for both viewing and economy. One edge of a a sheet of lead rubber can be attached, with the adhesive tape, across the width of a small cassette. In this position, it can move like the leaf of a book, allowing each half of the film to be exposed separately (Fig. 9.11).

Alternatively — as many manufactures of X-ray film have ceased to produce cassettes and film smaller than 18 × 24 cm — careful positioning, with good diaphragms or collimating cylinders, will allow two exposures on one film without overlapping or fogging. The lead rubber thus becomes unnecessary (Fig. 9.12).

9.3   AUXILIARY VIEWS TAKEN WITHOUT A GRID

9.3.1   Soft tissue techniques to demonstrate foreign bodies

In some cases of trauma it may be necessary to diagnose and localize fragments of teeth or other foreign bodies embedded in the facial soft tissue. The most usual instances will be in the upper and lower lip.

All these auxiliary views should be taken with a low kilovoltage and a greatly reduced milliamperage in order to demonstrate the foreign body.

- At normal exposures small fragments can easily be over-penetrated and blacked out on the film.

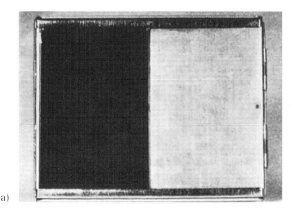

(a)

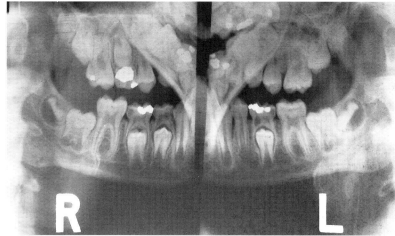

(b)

Fig. 9.11 (a) Cassette with sheet of lead hinged down the centre; (b) oblique lateral views of a 10-year-old child, taken on the cassette.

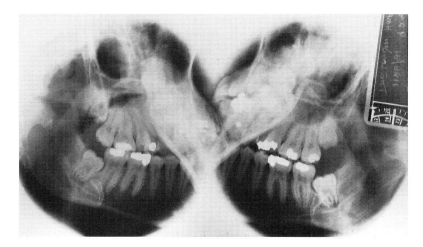

Fig. 9.12 Two exposures, taken on one 18 × 24 cm film, demonstrating mesioangular impacted lower wisdom teeth and unerupted upper third molars.

- Two views should be taken in planes at right angles to each other.

1. *Anterior view*

Place an 1–0 intra-oral film buccally, inside the lip, and angle the X-ray beam to throw the suspected area on to the film. There is obviously a limit to the placement of the film into the labial sulcus and an angulation of 10°, or even 20°, is acceptable (Fig. 9.13(a)).

2. *True lateral*

Place an occlusal film parallel to the sagittal plane, behind the area to be examined, and bring the X-ray beam at right angles to the film (Figs 9.13(b) and 9.14).

3. *Occlusal projection*

If the foreign body is in the lower lip, not in the midline, then an occlusal will also give another view at right angles, without the superimposition of the mandible.

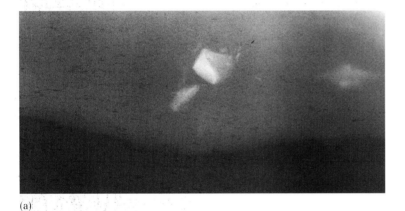

(a)

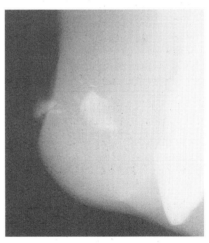

(b)

Fig. 9.13   Tooth fragments in upper lip: (a) film placed in the labial sulcus; (b) true lateral.

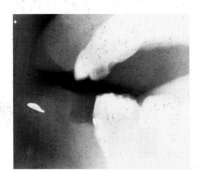

Fig. 9.14   Soft tissue true lateral showing foreign body in lower lip.

- Place the film in the occlusal plane, pushing it well out into the cheek.
- Centre the X-ray beam carefully, so that the central ray is directed at 90° to the film.

If the foreign body is in the upper cheek, push the film well out and direct the beam downwards on to the film.

It is sometimes possible to demonstrate a calculus in the parotid salivary duct with this technique, directing the beam along the line of the duct and angling from behind, to throw the image of any stone forwards on to the film (See Fig. 13.1(c)).

4. Rotated postero-anterior views
These are used to demonstrate:

- a foreign body in the lateral side of the face
- calculi in the parotid gland.

A non-screen film or cassette of 18×24 cm (or larger if available) is placed vertically in front of the patient's face, with the forehead and nose resting against it. (Ideally, a film stand should be used, but a co-operative patient may hold the film against a wall or stable vertical surface.)

- The sagittal plane is vertical and the orbital-meatal line is horizontal.
- Rotate the head 10° away from the affected side and the direct the central beam tangentially along the line of the ramus (Fig. 9.15).

9.3.2 The nasal bones

1. True lateral
The patient holds the film (occlusal or 18×24 cm cassette) parallel to the sagittal plane, behind the base of the nose.

- Direct the X-ray beam at right angles to the film, centring over nose (Fig. 9.16).

2. Supero-inferior
An occlusal film is placed in the mouth with two-thirds of the film projecting outside teeth.

- The X-ray beam is centred along the median plane of the head, above the frontal eminence, and directed perpendicularly to the plane of the film. It is important to give the appropriate exposure factors, depending upon whether screen or non-screen (occlusal) film is used.

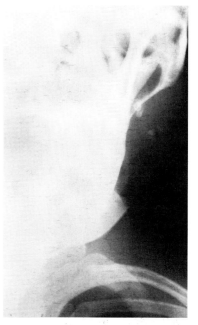

Fig. 9.15 Rotated postero-anterior with 10° rotation, with soft tissue exposure. This radiograph shows phleboliths in the cheek.

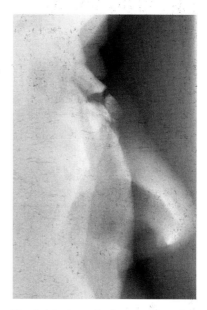

Fig. 9.16 Lateral soft tissue projection of nasal region to show fractured nasal bones.

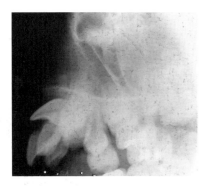

Fig. 9.17   Occlusal film used for lateral view of the maxilla. Position of unerupted anterior teeth can be seen.

9.3.3   True lateral of the maxilla

In dental practice, when cephalometry is not available, a useful lateral view of the maxilla may be obtained with a low-powered dental apparatus. This view, incorporated with an upper occlusal, will help localize supernumaries and unerupted canines.

- The patient holds an occlusal or 18 × 24 cm film parallel to the sagittal plane. It is suggested that the patient's thumb should steady the lower border, while the fingers press the posterior region of the film against the ascending ramus area. In this way, the film can remain in the correct plane, parallel to the median line of the face.
- The X-ray beam is horizontal and centred over the anterior portion of the maxilla.

If an occlusal film is taken, the exposure factors are twice those normally given for a central anterior upper **occlusal** (Fig. 9.17).

With 18 × 24 cm non-screen or cassette films, the exposure factors will be similar to those for oblique laterals.

Tangential view of maxilla
This view is useful to confirm buccally placed canines. The patient holds an occlusal film against the maxilla in the premolar region — care should be taken to ensure that the film is anterior enough to demonstrate the canine.

The X-ray beam is directed tangentially to the maxilla where the tooth can be palpated, and is horizontal, centred over the canine.

The exposure factors are similar to those normally given for anterior upper occlusals.

Lateral of mandible
This view can help to demonstrate the position of a tooth or cyst in the midline. The patient holds the film parallel to the sagittal plane behind the anterior region of the mandible.

The X-ray beam is horizontal and at right angles to the film.

The central ray is centred over the symphysis menti.

Normal exposure factors are given for the position of a tooth, when using either an occlusal or a cassette film.

Lower exposure factors are given for a cyst (Fig. 9.18).

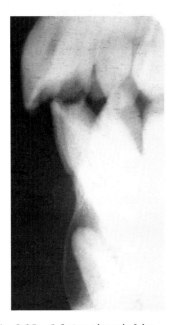

Fig. 9.18   Soft tissue lateral of the mandible demonstrating unerupted tooth associated with a dentigerous cyst in the incisor region. (See also Fig. 9.9 and Fig. 8.4, p. 137.)

FURTHER READING AND REFERENCES

Brocklebank, L. (1997). *Dental radiology: understanding the X-ray Image*. Oxford University Press, Oxford.

Waite, E. (1996). *Essentials of dental radiography and radiology* (2nd edn). Churchill Livingstone, London.

Haring, J.L. and Lind, L.J. (1996). *Dental radiography: principles and techniques.* W.B. Saunders and Co., Philadelphia.

Miles, D.A. (1989). *Radiographic imaging for dental auxiliaries.* W.B. Saunders and Co., Philadelphia.

Key points

Soft tissues
1. Reduce exposure factors
2. Two views at right angles
   — intra-oral or occlusal, lip or cheek
   — true lateral

Rotated postero-anterior of facial bones

For position of buccally placed teeth and cysts either
1. Rotate head 10° away from affected side
   — X-ray beam tangential
   or
2. True lateral or tangential auxiliary views

Rotate appropriate area to film, and direct X-ray beam at 90° to film

10 Extra-oral radiography: II Radiography of the facial bones

10.1 INTRODUCTION

This chapter covers radiography of the facial bones usually undertaken in hospital maxillofacial units.

Before carrying out any form of skull or facial bone radiography, the patient must remove all opaque accessories which could be superimposed over the bony structures, obscuring pathology and radiological diagnosis. Such objects would include ear-rings and metal necklaces and, of course, dentures and removable orthodontic appliances.

Due to the density of the skull, intensifying screens must be used to cut down the amount of radiation to the patient and, consequently, to reduce the scattered radiation. Nevertheless, there will still be some scattered radiation which will cause a general fogging of the film and, ideally, secondary radiation grids should be used.

Grids

Grids are composed of a series of thin lead slats which are placed with the long axis at right angles to the direction of the grid. The slats are separated by a radiotranslucent material. In this way, only those rays travelling in the direction of the slats can reach the film, whereas those that are scattered at different angles are absorbed by the lead (Fig. 10.1(a)). Good stationary grids have fine lines and a large number of slats to the centimetre, which make them almost invisible. They are placed immediately in front of the film.

Though grids minimize scattered radiation and improve the quality of the resultant radiograph, they will also remove some of the primary radiation and, thus, require the radiation exposure to be increased.

The focus–film distance

The focus–film distance is of paramount importance, with the use of a suitable diaphragm or collimating device (see p. 20) to confine the

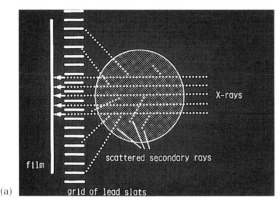
(a)

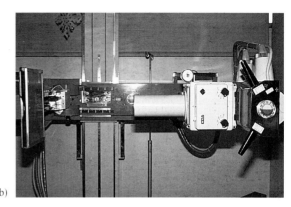
(b)

Fig. 10.1   (a) Diagrammatic presentation of the absorption of secondary irradiation by use of a grid; (b) dedicated skull unit demonstrating collimating device.

X-ray beam to the more central and parallel rays (Fig. 10.1(b)). The longer the focus–film distance, the less the enlargement of the image and the sharper the bone detail.

A dedicated skull unit with integral grid is often used for skull and facial bone work, since this is designed especially so that high-quality images can be achieved (see Fig. 10.1(b)). These usually have a focus–film distance of 100–120 cm.

An important part of these techniques is the immobilization of the head. If for any reason a dedicated skull unit is not used, headbands, made with self-adhesive Velcro, could be a useful adjunct, and can be adapted to any vertical cassette stand.

Position of the patient

In this chapter, the techniques are described with the patient sitting erect. The positions will be referred to in terms relating to the planes of the body (that is, sagittal, and coronal) as well as the relevant baselines of the skull.

- The radiographic baseline for the facial bones is the orbital-metal line, which extends from the external auditory meatus to the outer canthus of the eye ('OM line').
- The infra-orbital line runs across the face from one infra-orbital margin to the other.
- The Frankfort plane extends from the top of the tragus of the ear to the lower orbital margin.

In general, the projections are named according to the direction of the X-ray beam entering the head, for example, postero-anterior, and indicating the angle of the beam to the film, for example, 30° occipitomental.

Key points

- All opaque accessories to be removed from head and neck
- Intensifying screens to be used
- Ideally secondary radiation grid to be used
- Dedicated skull unit is often used

Patient positioned in terms of the planes of the body and relevant baselines of the skull

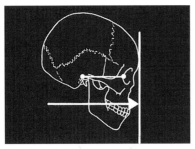

(a)

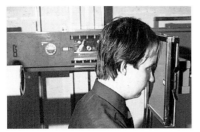

(b)

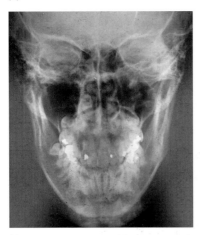

(c)

Fig. 10.2   (a) Diagram to demonstrate the position of the head for a postero-anterior projection of the facial bones; (b) a patient positioned for this view; (c) actual poster-anterior view. Note the superimposition of bony structures over the condyle region.

10.2   POSTERO-ANTERIOR TECHNIQUES

10.2.1   Postero-anterior (PA)

This projection is taken to demonstrate:

(1) fractures of the body, angle, or ramus of the mandible, and displacement of fractures, especially in a medio-lateral direction;

(2) Le Fort type I fracture of the middle third of the face;

(3) gross displacement of the zygomatic buttress;

(4) displacement of teeth in alveolar fractures;

(5) cysts or tumours in the rami, showing expansion of the bone in a medio-lateral direction;

(6) deformity of the mandible or the maxillofacial area.

Position of head

● Patient faces the film and the grid.
● *OM line*: parallel to the floor and perpendicular to the film.
● *Sagittal plane*: vertical and perpendicular to the film.
● *X-ray beam*: parallel to the floor.
● *Centring point*: mid-point of the X-ray beam centres over the mid-point of the ramus of the mandible to include the symphysis mentis and the temporomandibular joints

(Fig. 10.2)

10.2.2   Postero-anterior 15–20° (sometimes called a 'reverse townes')

This projection is taken to demonstrate:

(1) the neck and head of the condyles in a postero-anterior direction;

(2) fractures of the neck of the condyle.

Position of head

● Patient faces the film.
● *OM line*: horizontal and perpendicular to the film.
● *Sagittal plane*: vertical
● *X-ray beam*: 15°–20° upwards to the head.
● *Centring point*: at the level of the heads of the condyles of the jaw, in the midline. This view should be performed with the patient's mouth open. However, if there is a fracture of the condyles, this is not always possible

(Fig. 10.3)

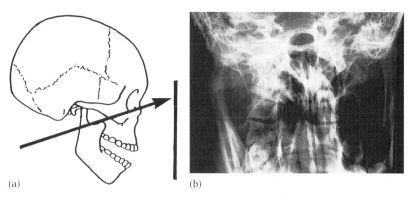

Fig. 10.3 (a) Diagram of the position for the postero-anterior, with upward angle of the X-ray tube; (b) postero-anterior view to demonstrate the neck of the condyles. Note the fracture of the right condyle.

This view may be done in the antero-posterior position (Fig. 10.4).

10.2.3   Occipitomental (OM)

This projection is taken to demonstrate:

(1) diagnosis of pathological conditions affecting the air sinuses, especially the maxillary antra, for example, tumours, cysts, fluid levels;

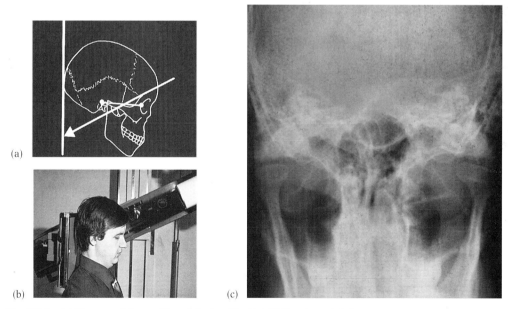

Fig. 10.4 (a) Diagram of the position of the head for the 30° fronto-occipital (Townes) projection; (b) a patient positioned for the Townes view; (c) Townes view, with the mouth open, to demonstrate shape of the condylar heads in the sagittal plane.

(2) fractures of the maxillofacial region, for example, Le Fort I, II, and III, the zygomatic region, orbits.

Position of head

- Patient faces film and grid.
- *OM line*: 45° to floor so that the petrous bones will be demonstrated below the maxillary sinuses.
- *Sagittal plane*: vertical and perpendicular to the film.
- *X-ray beam*: parallel to the floor and perpendicular to the film. (If the X-ray beam is not parallel to the floor, a fluid level in the sinuses will not be demonstrated.)
- *Centring point*: 5 cm above the occipital protuberance.

(Fig. 10.5)

This view must not project the petrous bones over the maxillary sinuses. So, the angle of the X-ray beam may need to vary according to individual anatomical configurations or owing to poor patient co-operation when unable to raise their chin sufficiently.

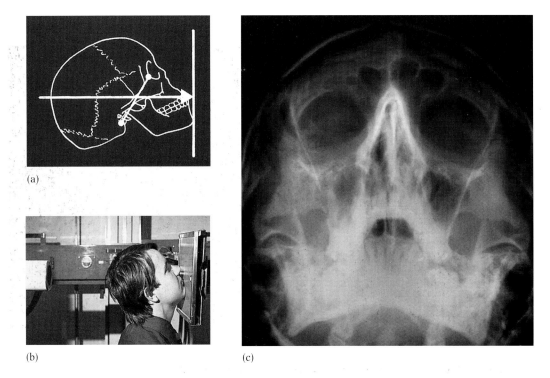

(a)

(b)

(c)

Fig. 10.5 (a) Diagram for the position of the head for the occipitomental projection; (b) a patient positioned for this view; (c) occipitomental view to demonstrate fractures of the right zygomatico-maxillary complex.

10.2.4   30° occipitomental (30° OM)

This projection demonstrates the

(1) fractures of the middle third of the face, including the orbital floor;
(2) a blow out fracture of the orbit;
(3) fractures of the zygomatic arches.

Position of head

- Patient faces the film and grid.
- *OM line*: 45° to the floor.
- *Sagittal plane*: vertical and perpendicular to the film.
- *X-ray beam*: 30° downward to the floor.
- *Centring point*: Mid-point of X-ray beam to emerge at the lower orbital margin

(Fig. 10.6)

Key points

- For postero-anterior views the patient sits facing the film
- Postero-anterior of jaws demonstrate fractures of the ramus, body or angle of the mandible
- P.A. 15–20° demonstrates the condyles
- O.M. demonstrates fractures and pathology of the middle third of the face
- O.M. 30° demonstrates floor of the orbits and zygomas

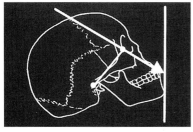

(a)

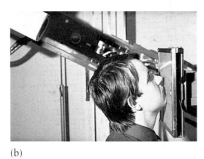

(b)

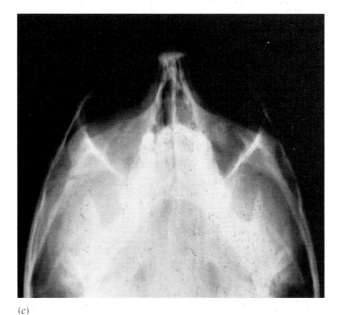

(c)

Fig. 10.6   (a) Diagram for the position of the head for the 30° occipitomental projection; (b) a patient positioned for this view; (c) 30° occipitomental view to demonstrate the fracture patterns in the floor of the orbit and on the inferior surface of the zygomatic arch.

10.3   ANTERO-POSTERIOR (AP)
TECHNIQUES

10.3.1   Submentovertical (SMV)

This projection is taken to demonstrate:

(1) fractures of the zygomatic arches;

(2) the base of the skull;

(3) the angle of inclination of the head of the condyle from the coronal plane to assess if a true AP projection is necessary.

This projection may be used as part of osteotomy work with lateral and postero-anterior cephalometric projections.

Position of head
The patient leans backwards with the vertex of the head against the film. With a skull table, the patient can lean back to a reasonable extent and the tube position can be compensated as appropriate.

- *OM line*: vertical as possible.
- *Coronal plane*: parallel to the film.
- *Sagittal plane*: perpendicular to the film.
- *X-ray beam*: 90° to OM line.
- *Centring point*: in the median plane, 5 cm above the angles of the mandible.

(Fig. 10.7(a))

Fractures of the zygomatic arches

To demonstrate these, it is usually necessary to reduce the exposure factors, most commonly the kilovoltage, with or without a grid. Whilst it is important not to black out the zygomatic arches, it is also essential that there is enough penetration of the X-ray beam to assess that the patient is correctly positioned, with the sagittal plane vertical.

Position of head

- *Patient, as above.*
- *X-ray beam*: 90° to zygomatic arch or 90–100° to OM line.
- *Centring point*: in the median plane, midway between the angles of the mandible. See Figs 10.7(a), (b), and (c).

Even a small amount of rotation can give the appearance of a depressed zygomatic arch. If the patient has a very depressed fracture of one zygomatic arch, it may be necessary to rotate away from that side.

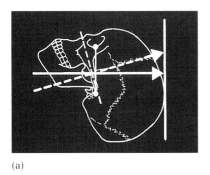

(a)

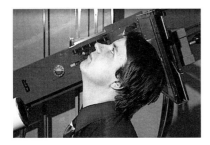

(b)

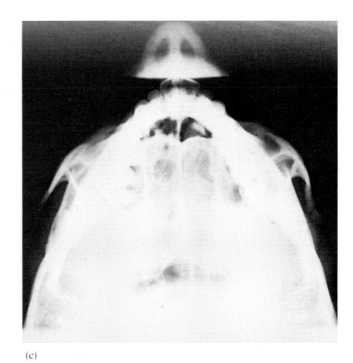

(c)

Fig. 10.7   (a) Diagram for the position of the head for the submentovertical projection; (b) a patient positioned for the submentovertical view to demonstrate the zygomatic arches; (c) submentovertical soft tissue exposure to demonstrate a depressed fracture of the left zygoma.

10.4   LATERAL TECHNIQUES

10.4.1   **Lateral for the facial bones and sinuses**

This projection is taken to demonstrate:

(1) backward displacement of fractures of the middle third of the facial bones, as in Le Fort I, II, and III;

(2) integrity or otherwise of the posterior walls of the antra;

(3) perforations of the hard palate;

(4) a foreign body in the airway.

Position of head

• Patient sits with the side under examination closest to the film.
• *Sagittal plane*: parallel to the film and grid.
• *Infra-orbital line*: 90° to the film.

Key points

• Patients for antero-posterior views sit with the back of the head next to the film.
• SMV demonstrates both the zygomas and the base of skull
• Reduce exposures for zygomatic arches
• Lateral views can be for both the facial bones and the vault of the skull

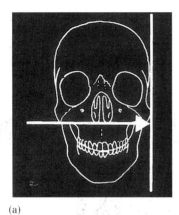

(a)

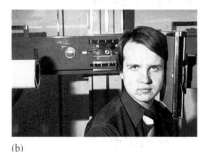

(b)

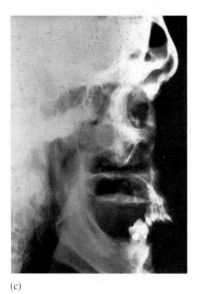

(c)

Fig. 10.8   (a) Diagram for the position of the head for lateral view of the facial bones; (b) a patient positioned for this view; (c) lateral of the facial bones confirming fluid level in a frontal sinus.

- *X-ray beam*: parallel to the floor and perpendicular to the film.
- *Centring point*: 1 cm below the outer canthus of the eye, to include the facial bones and the sinuses, Fig. 10.8.

10.4.2   Vault of the skull

This view is taken to demonstrate:

(1) fractures of the cranium;

(2) pathology, for example, Paget's disease (Fig. 10.9).

Position of head

- Patient positioned as for the facial bones.
- *X-ray beam*: parallel to the floor.
- *Centring point*: midway between the glabella and the external occipito-protuberance.

Radiographers, please note: the term 'lateral skull', to dentists, can indicate a lateral facial bones projection taken in a cephalostat.

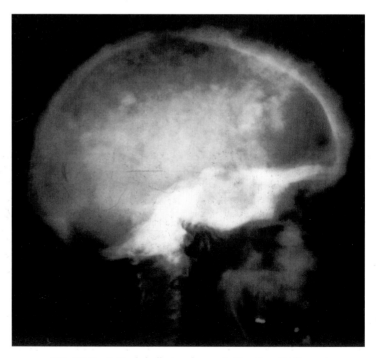

Fig. 10.9   Lateral skull view demonstrating Paget's disease.

10.5   TEMPOROMANDIBULAR JOINTS (TMJ)

10.5.1   Lateral oblique 25°/ transcranial

This view is taken to demonstrate:

(1) destruction of the condyle due to osteoarthritis;

(2) the degree of movement of the joint.

Position of head

- Patient sits with whichever side is under examination, nearest the film.
- *Sagittal plane*: parallel with the film.
- *Infra-orbital line*: 90° to the film.
- *X-ray beam*: 25° to the floor.
- *Centring point*: 5 cm above the tragus of the ear remote from the film, so that the mid-point of the beam emerges at the joint under examination.

(Fig. 10.10)

When the movement of the joints is to be demonstrated, two images are always taken — one with the mouth open, one closed. Both sides are taken for comparison.

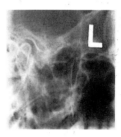

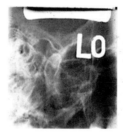

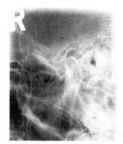

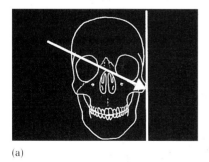

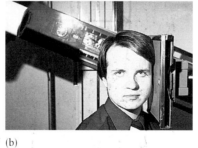

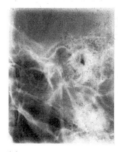

(a)   (b)   (c)

Fig. 10.10   (a) Diagram for the position of the head to show the temporomandibular joints (TMJ); (b) a patient positioned for transcranial projection of TMJ; (c) temporomandibular joints showing each side open and closed. The left condyle has moved much more than the right.

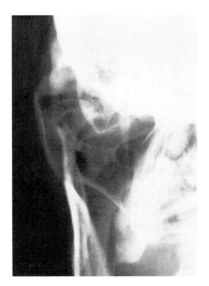

Fig. 10.11 An antero-posterior projection of the head of the condyle. The head is rotated about 10° towards the film, with the mouth open. Some erosion of the head of the condyle can be seen.

10.5.2　Transorbital projection

This projection is taken to demonstrate the head of the condyle in the antero-posterior position.

Position of head
The patient sits facing the X-ray tube, if possible, with the mouth open. The head is rotated towards the film until the ramus is 90° to it. This is an angle of about 10° and will vary with the inclination of the glenoid fossa to the coronal plane. This inclination would be demonstrated in an SMV projection.

- *OM line*: parallel to the floor and perpendicular to the film.
- *X-ray beam*: 20° to the floor, through the orbit.
- *Centring point*: to the joint under examination.
(Fig. 10.11).

The head could be in the postero-anterior position and the X-ray beam directed from below (similar to the reverse Townes projection) and centred up to the joint under examination.

10.5.3　Transpharyngeal view of head of condyle (Macqueen–Dell)

This projection will demonstrate:

(1) the head and neck of the condyles;

(2) hyper- or hypoplasia of the condylar head;

(3) a grossly displaced fracture of the condyle;

The condyles are best demonstrated with the mouth in the open position, when the head is out of the glenoid fossa.

The anode–film distance

The collimating device should be replaced by a diaphragm, to limit the field of irradiation to a practical minimum 4–6 cm diameter.

The anode–film distance, is kept to the minimum permissible in the Code of Practice (ICRP 1985), and should be performed on apparatus operating between 65–75 kVp to keep the skin dose down to a minimum. The use of standard intensifying or rare-earth screens, rather than the finer ones used in oblique laterals will also help keep the radiation dose as low as possible.

Key points

- Lateral-oblique 25° films are performed with the patients mouth open and closed
- Both sides are done for comparison
- Demonstrates the degree of movement of the joint as well as pathology
- Transpharyngeals are done with the patient in the dental chair
- Demonstrates the head and neck of the condyles.

Position of the patient

The patient sits in the dental chair, holding the film (the thumb supports the lower border, and the fingers hold the film against the external auditory meatus). The film is parallel with the sagittal plane and the X-ray beam is directed 5° up and 5° backwards towards the joint. Centring must be very accurate and is achieved by placing the joint, if possible with the mouth open, in the centre of the film, and centring to that point.

As with oblique laterals, both sides may be demonstrated on one 18 × 24 cm film. Due to the inevitable high radiation dosage, the authors recommend that this technique should only be undertaken in maxillofacial units, by experienced radiographers (Fig. 10.12).

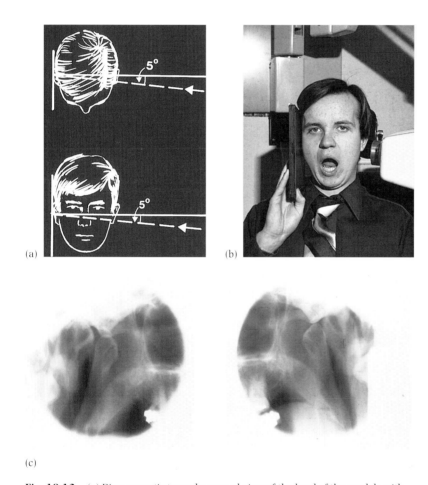

(a)

(b)

(c)

Fig. 10.12 (a) Diagrammatic transpharyngeal view of the head of the condyle with the central ray directed 5° up and 5° backwards, towards the condyle to be examined; (b) a patient positioned for transpharyngeal view; (c) transpharyngeal views of the right and left condyles. A small erosion of the head of the right condyle is demonstrated.

10.5.4   Discussion

There are many techniques advocated to demonstrate the movement of the temporomandibular joint and to show changes in the bony contour of the head of the condyle, but due to anatomical variation between patients, it is very difficult to recommend absolute techniques. It is often possible to obtain perfect results on one patient, and to fail miserably to demonstrate the joint at all on the next patient. This is due to many functional factors. If the head of the condyle is to be demonstrated, and the patient can open his or her mouth, then the transpharyngeal view is generally the easiest to achieve and will give the most satisfactory view of the head of the condyle, for bony erosions. Due to its relatively high radiation dose (5.7 mSv), it should be prescribed specifically and with caution, when other views prove to be inconclusive for diagnosis.

It is only possible to demonstrate the head of the condyle in the true lateral projection within the glenoid fossa, with the aid of information gained from an axial projection. This also applies when a true AP projection is necessary. It is also possible to demonstrate the head of the condyle and its movement with rotational tomographic apparatus. This can be undertaken in general practice, but only with very specific instruction.

Tomography of the joints can be performed in the AP and lateral projections, using either conventional tomography equipment or dedicated cranio-maxillofacial imaging equipment, for example, Scanora, Tomax, or Commcat. The true AP views are more difficult to achieve, and the Townes or reverse Townes view, with the mouth open, gives a good comparative projection.

Overall, the choice of views will depend upon the skill of the operator and conformity of the patient.

10.6   CEPHALOMETRY

This is the technique used to study maxillofacial growth and facial deformity, with measurements and comparisons of specific points taken by the orthodontist and the maxillofacial surgeon.

The essential quality of cephalometry is that the resultant radiographs are comparable and reproducible. A serial study can be undertaken to assess the growth and development of the facial skeleton, and to analyse the results of active orthodontic treatment or corrective surgical procedures in facial abnormalities.

The head must be immobilized in a special head holder called a 'cephalostat' or 'craniostat'. There are different types of cephalostat, but they all embody the same basic principles: two long arms enclose the head; they are usually made of plastic and are controlled by a framework of metal; and they are directed from above or behind, adjusting to fit different widths of head. The head is fixed by means of two small, horizontal pegs at the end of the localizing arms, which are introduced into the external auditory meatus. Usually, these pegs include some metal, to determine the accuracy of this technique — including the stability of the cephalostat and the alignment of the X-ray beam – for example, two rings to be superimposed, or a dot within a ring. (Fig. 10.13)

The focus–film distance must be 1.5–1.8 m to achieve a nearly parallel X-ray beam. The X-ray tube should be in a fixed position, so that the central ray is exactly centred to the external auditory meatus and the cephalostat.

A movable aluminium wedge is attached to the cephalostat to attenuate the X-rays reaching the anterior portion of the image and to produce a soft tissue outline of the face as well as the facial bones. This wedge can be placed in front of the patient, which can help to lessen the radiation dose to the eyes. Some cephalostats have a wedge on the tube itself, with the added advantage that there will be no lines of demarcation (for example, Siemens' Orthophos CD and Gendex' Orthoralix SD ceph) (Fig. 10.14).

It is also possible to place a wedge between the patient and the film. This position of the wedge has the disadvantage of projecting a sharp line of demarcation, and can obscure some of the anterior specific tracing landmarks. Another way of obtaining both hard and soft tissue images with one exposure is by placing a fast and slow speed film into the same cassette.

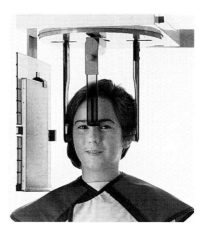

Fig. 10.13   Position of a patient for a lateral cephalometric skull view.

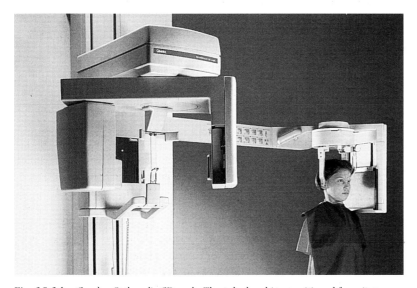

Fig. 10.14   Gendex Orthoralix SD ceph. The tube head is repositioned from its dental panoramic programme. The filter is adjustable at the tube head.

In all methods, it must be possible to vary the filter to the size and shape of the patient's contour. The cephalostat should include a film holder, and a stationary grid may be used.

There is equipment that allows both dental panoramic tomography and cephalometry. The focus-film distance is not as long as already stated, and the filter is placed in the tube head. As in all cephalometry, it is important that the magnification remains the same for each radiograph, so that there is standardization and reproducibility.

Recent developments in technology now enable images to be produced using a special digital sensor, and viewed and measured on a computer screen, for example, Siemens' Orthophos DS Ceph. The images can then be archived on disk, so there is no need for film processing or a darkroom. (See Chapter 7.)

10.6.1 Lateral cephalometric view

This view will demonstrate:

(1) the relationship of the soft to hard tissue of the face;
(2) the position of the teeth in relationship to each other and to the hard tissues and bony structures;
(3) the skeletal pattern;
(4) the tracing and scanning points necessary for orthodontic assessment.

(Fig. 10.15)

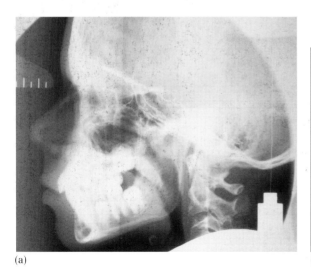
(a)

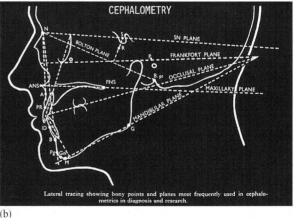
(b)

Fig. 10.15 (a) Cephalometric lateral view of the facial bones — an aluminium wedge was used to show the soft tissue outline; (b) a cephalometric tracing showing the main cephalometric planes, angles and points.

Position of the patient

The patient is placed in the cephalostat, with the ear pieces positioned into the EAMs.

The aluminium wedge is placed so that the thin edge is aligned to protect the eye as much as possible, whilst still demonstrating the required soft tissue outline. The teeth must be in centric occlusion, that is, with back teeth together. Some patients find this difficult and may need help.

- *Frankfort plane*: horizontal (supratragal notch to the lower border of the orbit).
- *Sagittal plane*: parallel to the film.
- *X-ray beam*: automatically pre-set to be horizontal.
- *Centring point*: automatically pre-set to pass through both EAMs.
- *Anode–film distance*: 180 cm. (This is the anode-film distance necessary to achieve a true parallel beam of X-rays.)

In equipment that offers combined dental panoramic tomography and cephalometry, the anode–film distance is reduced because of the power of the apparatus, combined with spatial considerations (Fig. 10.16).

10.6.2   Postero-anterior cephalometric view

Most cephalostats can be rotated through 90°, and then a postero-anterior position undertaken. This projection will demonstrate:

(1) the position of unerupted canines;

(2) asymmetry of the facial bones;

(3) assessment of jaws, pre- and post-operative orthognathic surgery.

Position of patient

The head should be positioned in exactly the same way as for the lateral projection. Thus, two views can be achieved at right angles to each other.

Rotate the cephalostat through 90° and position the patient, with the ear pieces, into the EAMs. The patient occludes on to the back teeth.

- *Sagittal plane*: perpendicular to the film.
- *Coronal plane*: parallel to the film.
- *Frankfort plane*: perpendicular to the film.
- *X-ray beam*: automatically pre-set to be horizontal.
- *Centring point*: in the midline, at the level of the EAMs.
- Anode–film distance: 180 cm.

(Fig. 10.17)

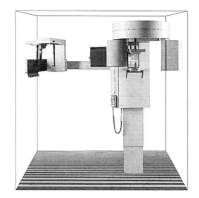

Fig. 10.16 Siemens Orthophos CD. There is combined dental panoramic tomography and cephalometry in this compact piece of equipment.

Key points

- Cephalometry studies facial growth and deformity
- The radiographs must be standarised and reproducable
- The head is immobilised in a special head holder
- There must be an almost parallel X-ray beam to reduce the magnification factor
- Lateral radiographs must include a soft tissue outline of the face
- P.A. cephs are performed to demonstrate asymmetry of the face
- The patient must occlude on the back teeth

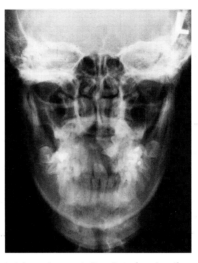

Fig. 10.17   Cephalometric postero-anterior view showing three unerupted teeth on the left side of the maxilla. The height and relationship of the teeth to the midline and floor of the nose is clearly seen.

REFERENCES AND FURTHER READING

Browne, R.M., Edmondson, H.D., and Rout, P.G. (1995). *A radiological atlas of diseases of the teeth and jaws.* Mosby Wolfe.

Goaz, P.W. and White, S.C. (1994). *Oral radiology — principles and interpretation* (3rd edn). Mosby Wolfe.

McIvor, J. (1986). *Dental and maxillo-facial radiology.* Churchill Livingstone, Edinburgh.

Stafne, E.C. (1985). *Oral roetgenographic diagnosis.* W.B. Saunders, Philadelphia.

Swallow, R.A. and Naylor, E.E. (1986) (ed) *Clarke's positioning in radiography* (11th edn) Heinemann, London.

Waites, E. (1996). *Essentials of dental radiography and radiology.* Churchill Livingstone, Edinburgh.

ICRP. (1985). *Approved code of Practice. The protection of persons against ionising radiation arising from any work activity. The Ionising Radiation Regulations.* HMSO, London.

11   Dental panoramic tomography

Tomography has been applied to dento-maxillofacial radiography in the form of rotational or panoramic radiography. The first experimental work was carried out in Japan, in 1933, but it was Professor Y.V. Paatero of Finland who succeeded in producing a practical application of the technique.

The tomographic film is not as clear as the stationary film, due to the blurring effect of the tissue above and below the selected layer. When the overlying layers are far enough away, they will be blurred out of perception, but the more adjacent structures will still cast their blurred shadow over the chosen focal cut (Fig. 11.1).

The requirements in the dental arches are different from linear tomography, where a layer within a mass is to be revealed. Dental panoramic tomography requires only that one side of the dental arch should not be superimposed upon the other, or the spine over the midline. Consequently, as much detail and clarity as possible is advantageous. A wide focal cut is to be desired. This is possible because there are no immediate bony structures adjacent to the dental arches, that is, it is a 'free zone' (Fig. 11.2). This allows for a

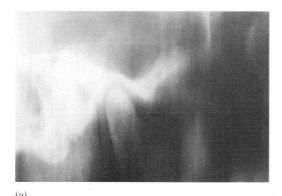
(a)

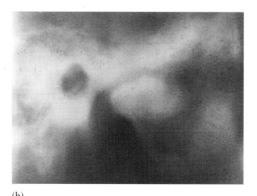
(b)

Fig. 11.1   These tomographic films demonstrate (a) a normal head of the condyle within the glenoid fossa; (b) a misshapen osteoarthritic and fibrous ankylosed head of the condyle.

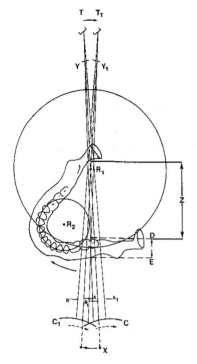

Fig. 11.2 Diagram demonstrating a small angle movement which produces a thick focal cut. This is possible because there is a free zone around the dental arches. T–T1 = movement of Z-ray beam during exposure angle; R1 = centre of rotation; D–E = zone of sharpness — focal cut; Z = free zone; F–F1 = movement of the film during exposure angle.

narrow exposure angle which produces a thicker focal cut, without the otherwise degrading effect of overlying blurring.

11.1   HISTORY OF DENTAL PANORAMIC TOMOGRAPHY

Professor Paatero went to the University of Washington in Seattle in 1950–51, where he evolved a prototype machine. It was as a result of his work with Dr Sydney Blackman, at the Royal Dental Hospital, London, that Watson's Ltd produced the first practical version of the 'Rotograph' in 1955. In this apparatus, Paatero used his original concept — a stationary X-ray source with the patient and film moving synchronously, the film anticlockwise and the head clockwise, at the same speed (Fig. 11.3). The head was placed in a craniostat and a film, attached to the holder, in the same shape as the mandible, was placed upon a concentric platform in a similar position to the centre of rotation as the dental arches in the craniostat. This meant that the effective speed of the film varied with its position from the centre of the platform.

Though revolutionary in concept, the Rotograph was not accurate enough in the canine and premolar region, as the approximal spaces did not lie on the radii from the centre of rotation. Paatero went back to the USA and started work on the further refinement of keeping the patient stationary, and moving the tube and film around the patient using two pivots. This principle is still used with the S.S. White Panorex, which was first available in 1959. There are two centres of rotation. The tube and film move in an are simulating the curve of one half of the dental arches. The patient is then moved so that a film of the other side may be taken (Figs 11.4(a) and (b) and 11.5). There is an overlap in the centre which may be cut out if required.

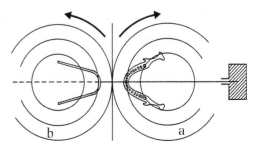

Fig. 11.3 The original Watson's Rotograph had a fixed tube head. The patient's mandible was positioned in a craniostat (a) and the film placed similarly on a concentric platform (b). They moved synchronously, in opposite directions.

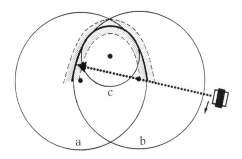

Fig. 11.4 Rotational tomography may be operated with two arcs of rotation (a and b), with the patient's position changed between each movement, for example, S.S. White's Panorex; or with three arcs of rotation (a, b, and c), using a continuous movement, for example, Siemen's Orthopantomograph.

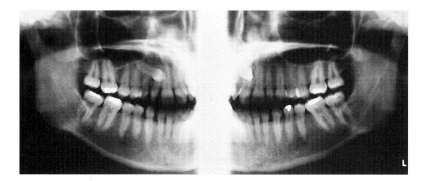

Fig. 11.5 This film (from a Panorex) shows how parallax can be used in the slit exposure, demonstrating a palatal upper right canine.

Afterwards, Paatero experimented with three rotational pivots, in order that the approximal spaces would coincide with the radii from the various centres of rotation — hence the name 'orth-radial-panoramic-tomography'. This was the basis of Siemens' Orthopantomography 1960 (see Fig. 11.4).

There is now apparatus available which continuously changes the centres of rotation between the three main pivots, so that the arc of the rotation takes an elliptical shape, to simulate the shape of the

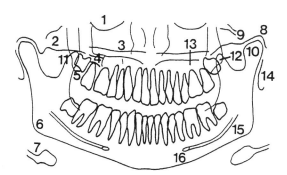

Fig. 11.6 Diagram of anatomical landmarks on the rotational tomograph: 1 = orbit, 2 = zygomatic arch, 3 = palate, 4 = septa in maxillary sinus, 5 = maxillary tuberosity, 6 = angle of mandible, 7 = hyoid bone, 8 = glenoid fossa, 9 = articular eminence, 10 = mandibular condyle, 11 = coronoid process, 12 = pterygoid plates, 13 = maxilla, 14 = ear lobe, 15 = mandibular canal, 16 = mental foramen.

Key points

- Dental panoramic Tomography was invented by Professor Paatero
- Dental panoramic tomography requires that one side of the dental arch is not superimposed on the other.
- The X-ray tube and film move equally and opposite around a pivot point
- This pivot point also moves, in an elliptical shape
- Modern dental panoramic equipment uses this movement
- The latest apparati also give a choice of different programs to image the jaw

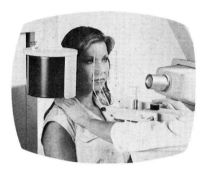

Fig. 11.7   Panelipse (General Electric Co.).

dental arches. This has the advantage that the X-radiation is no longer concentrated at two or three centres in the patient's head. Examples of this type of machine are:

- S.S. White's Panorex 2-continuous mode
- International General Electric's Panelipse (Figs 11.7 and 11.8)
- Monita's Panex (Fig. 11.9)
- Soredex's Cranex (Fig. 11.10)
- Siemens' OPG5 and 10 (Fig. 11.11), Orthophos, Orthophos 3, and Plus (Figs 11.12, 11.13, and 11.14)
- Planmecas' PM 2002 CC (Figs 11.15 and 11.16)
- Gendex Orthoralix S and SD2 (Fig. 11.17)

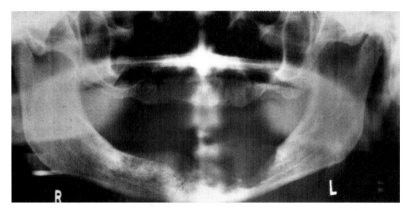

Fig. 11.8   Panelipse tomogram of edentulous patient to demonstrate an extensive malignant neoplasm eroding the upper border of the mandible on the left side.

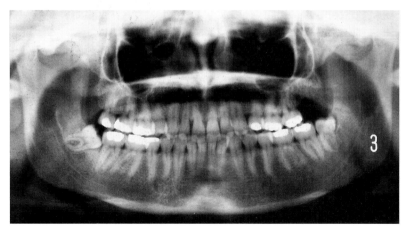

Fig. 11.9   Panex tomogram shows unerupted lower wisdom teeth.

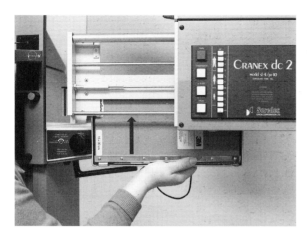

Fig. 11.10 Cranex dc 2 (Soredex) showing controls and the insertion of the flat cassette into this rotational tomographical apparatus.

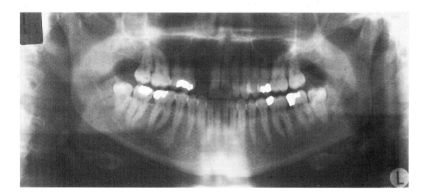

Fig. 11.11 This film (from an OPG10) demonstrates bilateral fractures of the mandible, through the base of the left condylar process, and the right angle. (Note the shadow of a necklace in the mid-line).

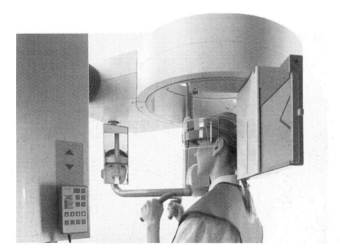

Fig. 11.12 Siemens' Orthophos.

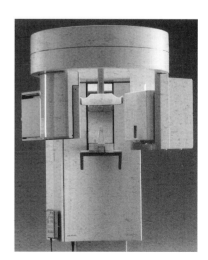

Fig. 11.13 Siemens' Orthophos Plus.

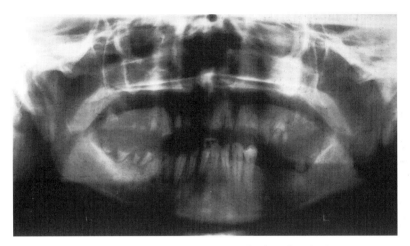

Fig. 11.14   Dental panoramic tomogram using Orthophos Plus, demonstrating rampant tooth decay in a young adult.

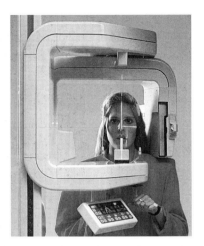

Fig. 11.15   PM 2002 CC (Panmeca).

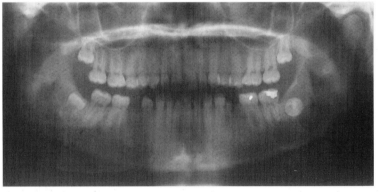

Fig. 11.16   Dental panoramic tomogram using Planmeca PM 2002 CC, demonstrating a large cystic area in the left angle and ramus of the mandible.

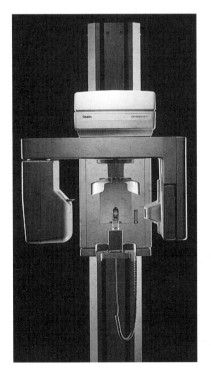

Fig. 11.17   Gendex Orthoralix S.

The latest apparatus give a choice of different programs which will not only provide rotational tomography for adults and children (with reduced area and dose), but also four views of the temporomandibular joints (TMJ), open and closed, antero-posterior (AP) and lateral tomograms of the TMJ (Fig. 11.18), as well as cross-sectional images of the jaw.

Palomex manufacture an apparatus, the Zonarc, where the patient is supine instead of vertical. It operates similarly for the dental arches as other rotational tomograph apparatus, and has other sophisticated options which include imaging for the middle third of the maxillofacial bones, the optic foramina, the inner ear, and TMJ (Fig. 11.19).

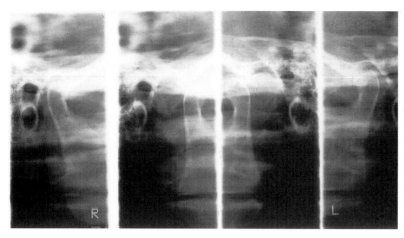

Fig. 11.18 Lateral TMJ with mouth open and closed on one film, using Orthophos CD.

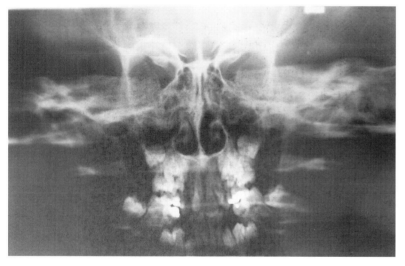

Fig. 11.19 Zonarc tomographic film giving maxillofacial mode. This tomogram shows a hemispherical soft tissue opacity projecting from the floor of the right orbit, consistent with the 'hanging drop sign' of an orbital 'blow out' fracture.

11.2   FORMATION OF THE FOCAL TROUGH

In all apparatus, it is essential that the X-ray beam should be confined by a narrow line diaphragm, and the film protected by a lead shield with a vertical aperture of about 1 cm.

The centres of rotation of pivot changes in rotational tomography are determined by the relative speed of the X-ray tube and film — the faster the speed and velocity ratio, the longer the radius. This is similar to multilayer tomography, where the differences in speed are minimal but allow planes as little as 1.5 mm apart to be projected separately.

In dental panoramic tomography, using the narrow beam of X-rays and shorter anode– object–film distances, the differences in speed are greater. When the velocity is slower and the radious is shorter, the exposure angle is wider and the focal cut is narrower. Consequently, the changing centres of rotation necessary to achieve the elliptical shape of the arches will result in differing depths to the focal cut — It is always narrower in the incisor and canine region (Fig. 11.20).

Every apparatus has its own pattern of movement, and the shape of the differing focal cuts is called the focal trough and is individual to each manufacturer.

In effect, rotational tomography is the composite of many small angle tomographs. In general, the focal trough will vary in depth between about 30 mm in the molar region to 5 mm in the anterior region. This presents difficulties, as the shape of the arches will vary between patients and, anteriorly, the trough may not be deep enough to contain the inclined incisors.

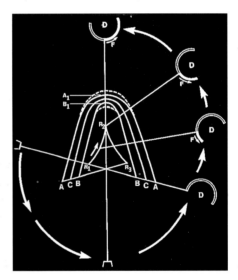

Fig. 11.20 The film (f) moves within the cassette drum (d). Its speed is synchronized with the narrow beam which is focused to the centre line. (c) The beam scans by continuously changing centres of rotation starting from R1. The borders (a) and (b) represents the limits of the object being scanned at the same velocity — the focal cut. As the beam reaches the forward centre of rotation, R2, with a shorter radius, it rotates to conform to the greater curvature of the anterior region of the dental arch. For the film and beam scan to remain synchronized, the relative velocity becomes slower. Thus, at the original border (a), the scan will be faster, and slower at (b), blurring the object. Consequently, the zone of sharpness (where the velocity remains constant) is narrowed in the anterior region A1–B1. The beam scan then continues to travel round to R3, reversing the effect.

- In fact, as the shape of the focal trough is constant, the quality of the resultant image will depend very largely on the skill of the operator in positioning the patient within it — so, the operator will profit by an understanding of this technique.

11.3 APPLICATIONS

(1) Assessment for presence and position of wisdom teeth;

(2) assessment of alveolar bone height in periodontal disease;

(3) assessment of both jaws prior to implants;

(4) assessment of both jaws prior to planing for dentures;

(5) to demonstrate fractures of the mandible;

(6) to demonstrate cysts, tumours, and other pathology in the mandible;

(7) for orthodontic assessment;

(8) to assess the extent of disease in young children.

11.4 OPERATION

In some apparatus, the film is placed in a curved metal cassette, for example, the OPG and Panex. The Panelipse has a flexible cassette, with flexible screens, which is wrapped around a drum. It is also possible to use a flat cassette, for example, the Cranex (see Fig. 11.10), PM 2002 CC (see Fig. 11.15), and Orthophos (see Fig. 11.12).

The film holder moves at the same speed as the X-ray tube, around the patient. The film and cassette are also moved rotationally or laterally, depending upon the apparatus, behind the lead shield. This allows for the continuous exposure of the film.

It is very important that the patient is positioned correctly in the focal trough. Each manufacturer will give exact operation instructions.

11.5 POSITIONING GUIDELINES

1. Dentures, neck chains, and ear-rings should be removed, as these obscure parts of the image (Fig. 11.21).

2. In some patients, the type of lead apron that fastens around the neck is not advised, as it can cast a shadow over the mid-line of

Key points

- All equipment has a narrow beam of X-rays
- The centres of rotation change
- Every piece of equipment has its own pattern of movement
- The shape of the differing focal cuts is called the image layer or the focal trough
- The focal trough is usually about 30 mm in the molar region and 10 mm in the incisor area
- The resultant image depends on the skill of the operator
- The patient must be positioned correctly

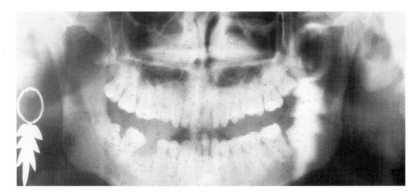

Fig. 11.21   This view (from a Panelipse) shows one large drop ear-ring casting a ghost image which is superimposed over an impacting third molar.

the film (Fig. 11.22). Lead aprons are used as a reassurance to the patient (see p. 70).

3.   The patient should be very erect, to keep the density around the spine to a minimum (Figs 11.23(a) and (b) and 11.24).

4.   The head should be carefully placed with the incisors edge to edge, with the use of a bite guide and a chin rest. In most skeletal patterns, this will then allow the incisors to be contained within the focal trough. The alatragal line is a guide in the positioning of the head and should usually incline about 5° downwards, The alternative is to have the Frankfurt plane parallel to the floor. This position will also minimize the hard palate shadow (see Fig. 11.23(b)).

(a)   If the ala-tragal line is down too much, the anterior region of the mandible will be out of focus and foreshortened. This position may, however, be useful for unerupted canines and the maxillary antra (Fig. 11.25).

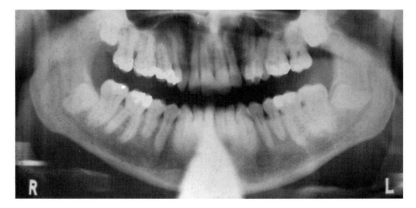

Fig. 11.22   Panelipse tomogram taken with a lead apron fastened behind the patient's neck, casting a triangular shadow over the lower incisor region.

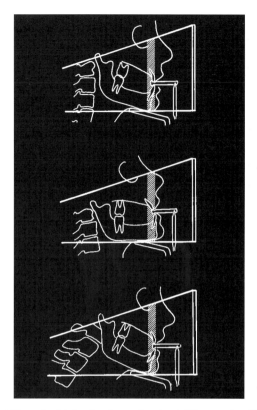

Fig. 11.23 (a) The patient is leaning forward and not sitting erect — the spine will cast a dense shadow over the incisor and canine regions; (b) correct positioning of the upper and lower incisors so that they lie within the focal trough; (c) incorrect positioning of the incisors. The maxillary incisors are moving out of the focal trough. The hard palate will cast a dense shadow. This position may demonstrate the anterior region of the mandible and the lower condyle.

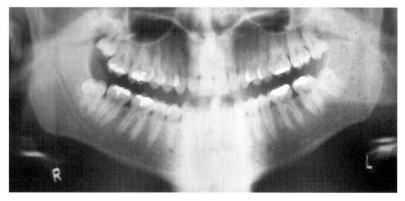

Fig. 11.24 Panelipse tomogram with the patient leaning forward and casting a dense spinal shadow over the anterior region of the jaws.

(b) If the ala-tragal line is inclined upwards, the maxilla is out of focus. This may bring the anterior position of the mandible entirely into the focal trough (see Figs 11.23 (c) and 11.26). Fractures of the mid-line can be demonstrated. Alternatively, if the head of the condyle on a large patient is to be seen together with the rest of the mandible, it allows the ramus to be tilted, and so lowers the level of the condyle.

5. There should be no rotation of the patient's head, as this will distort the image (Fig. 11.27).

6. If the patient's head is placed too far forward, there will be an overlap of the teeth in the body of the mandible, but the ramus and condyle will be well demonstrated (see Fig. 11.25).

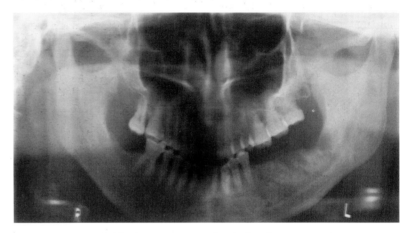

Fig. 11.25   Patient positioned with chin down too much.

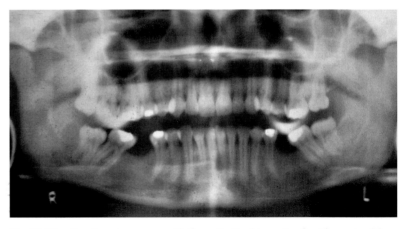

Fig. 11.26   Panelipse tomogram with the patient's chin up too far. The roots of the upper teeth are not in the focal trough. The hard palate casts a dense shadow. The patient's ear-rings are casting a secondary shadow over the upper molar regions.

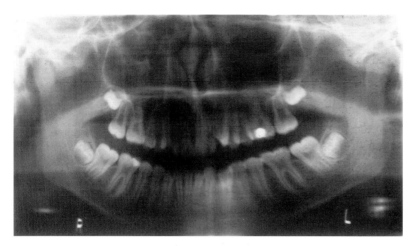

Fig. 11.27 Dental panoramic tomogram demonstrating distortion of the left side due to rotation of the patient's head.

7. If the patient's head is not placed far enough forward in position, then part of the ramus may be cut off and there is a 'pulled out' appearance of the teeth. Skilfully assessed, it can be useful in demonstrating interdental spaces (Fig. 11.28).

8. The patient should be instructed to close the lips around the bite guide. This places the tongue against the roof of the mouth and will help equalize the tissue densities.

9. In Panelipse, where the focal cut is adjusted for each patient, this *must* be done (Fig. 11.29).

10. In apparatus where the patient is positioned solely using the bite guide, care must be taken with patients who have very

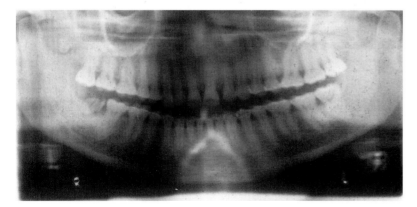

Fig. 11.28 Panelipse tomogram demonstrating the patient positioned too far from the film, making the incisors magnified. Note the artefact over the lower incisors due to failure to remove a necklace.

Key points

- All opaque items to be removed from the head and neck area
- Incisors placed edge to edge, slightly apart with the use of a bite guide
- The Frankfurt plane must be parallel to the floor
- No rotation of the head
- Patients lips to be closed around the bite guide
- For exact positioning and exposure factors, follow the manufacturers instructions

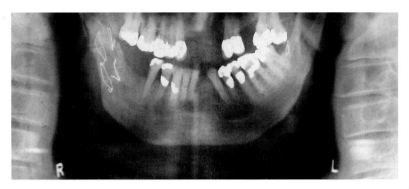

Fig. 11.29   In the Panelipse, the focal cut must be adjusted for each patient. This patient is, in effect, too far forward in the focal trough, with narrowing of the mandible.

proclined teeth. In these instances, to achieve the best results, though losing detail in the mid-line, the patient should be brought forward into the focal trough. In the Panorex 2, this is achieved by biting further forward on the peg or, in the Panelipse, by selecting a small focal cut. With apparatus such as the OPG 5 or 10, where the positioning is aided by vertical light lines, this problem is easier to overcome.

11. When the chin rest is lowered, it is sometimes possible to demonstrate fractures of the neck of the condyles. This will depend upon whether the condylar heads remain within the focal cut (Fig. 11.30).

12. On all modern dental panoramic equipment, there is the facility to image the TMJ, open and closed, in four separate exposures on one film. On the most up-to-date equipment, this is done by utilizing the programs set on the machine (see Fig. 11.18).

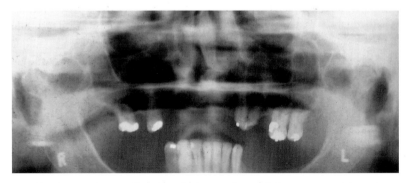

Fig. 11.30   Panelipse tomogram with chin rest lowered, demonstrating bilateral fractures of the condylar neck with overriding and loss of vertical height.

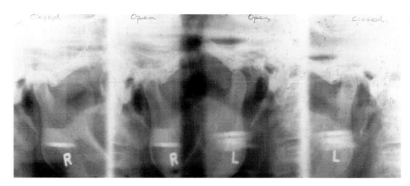

Fig. 11.31 Panelipse tomogram, taken with lowered chin rest and four separate timed exposures, demonstrating both TMJ in the open and closed positions. In this patient, the right condyle is barely moving and has lost some of its joint space. On the left, the head of the condyle is very far forward.

In apparatus such as the Panelipse, where the operation can be commenced from either side, the chin rest can be lowered and the condyle brought forward into the widest part of the focal trough. As the rotation commences, two separate, but timed, exposures are made in both positions of the condyle, on the side nearest the film. The tube and film are then reset and the procedure repeated for the other side (Fig. 11.31).

13. For exact positioning of the patient and for exposure factors, follow the manufacturer's instructions. Most apparatus function in the range of 8–15 mA 60–100 kVp. The exposure time during rotation is about 15–20 seconds.

11.6 ADVANTAGES

Dental panoramic radiography has become an important technique in dental radiography. An increasing number of general practitioners now include this apparatus with their X-ray equipment, for the following reasons:

1. It provides an overall survey of the teeth and facial bones with the minimum discomfort to, and the minimum co-operation from, the patient.

2. It allows for the assessment of the presence and position of unerupted teeth in orthodontic treatment.

3. It will demonstrate undiagnosed cysts, tumours, or buried teeth and roots in adults.

4. It enables the ascending rami, condyles, and coronoid processes to be seen together.

Key points

- There are many advantages for Dental panoramic tomography
- It demonstrates anatomy and pathology of the jaws
- The radiation dose is much less than full mouth periapicals
- The technique does have disadvantages, namely a lack of detail
- The anterior teeth are not always well demonstrated
- The equipment is relatively expensive
- Dental panoramic tomography should be prescribed with respect, not routinely

5. It will help in the assessment of the depth of the mandible, and the relationship of the inferior dental canal with the teeth or the alveolar margin.

6. It will demonstrate fractures of the mandible from the mid-line to the neck of the condyle, with less distortion than most oblique lateral views and, often, with less discomfort to the patient.

7. It will demonstrate periodontal disease in a general way, and allow individual intra-oral films to be kept to a minimum.

8. It will demonstrate an anterior view of the sinuses and floor of the nose.

9. The time taken to carry out this technique is short compared to a full mouth intra-oral examination, or even two oblique lateral views with complementary occlusal projections.

10. This technique is comparatively easy to undertake, in contrast to intra-oral techniques.

11. The radiation dose is approximately one third less than a full mouth intra-oral survey, depending on the speed of the intra-oral films and the film-screen combination used with the dental panoramic machine.

11.7   DISADVANTAGES

1. There is a lack of detail, as with all types of tomography.

2. There is also lack of detail and definition due to the use of intensifying screens.

3. The increased object–film distance causes enlargement of the image. This varies with each apparatus, for example, Panelipse 1.19, OPT10 1.23.

4. The density of the spine, particularly in short-necked patients, can cause lack of clarity in the central portion of the film.

5. Due to narrowness of the focal trough in the anterior region, it is often difficult to demonstrate the incisor and canine regions with adequate detail.

6. Patients with facial asymmetry, or who do not conform with the shape of the focal trough, will not project a satisfactory image.

7. Interstitial caries cannot be diagnosed, in most cases, owing to the lack of detail and the failure of this technique to demonstrate interdental spaces, particularly in the premolar region.

8. The object is elongated as there is an upward angulation of X-ray beam. The lingual or palatal aspect is projected relatively higher

than the buccal aspect. This can produce misleading images, for example, some lower third molars appear less impacted than they really are.

9. The cost of the equipment, which is supplementary to intra-oral techniques, is four to six times that of the regular dental apparatus. Some manufacturers combine the tube of the panoramic apparatus with a cephalostat, which will be economically advantageous, for example, Siemens' Orthophos CD and Planmeca PM 2002 CC Cephalometric (Fig. 11.32).

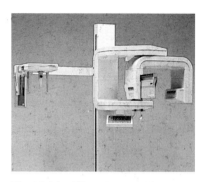

Fig. 11.32 Planmeca PM 2002 CC Cephalometric system.

11.8 CONCLUSION

Dental panoramic tomography has a very necessary and important place in dental radiography. It is used extensively in dental hospital X-ray departments, and is now found much more often in general dental practice. The radiation dosage is less than more extensive intra-oral surveys, and the panoramic view will give essential information before the treatment of new adult patients. It is a great asset for children, particularly during orthodontic treatment.

Before installing this apparatus, the practitioner must be sure that there is sufficient space and that the 1985 Ionising Radiation Regulations (IRR) are adhered to. The processing facilities may need upgrading or improved. (See Chapter 3.) To achieve consistent good results, the operator must have a basic knowledge of how the image is formed.

Dental panoramic tomography should be prescribed with respect, and not routinely before every course of treatment.

REFERENCES AND FURTHER READING

Chomenko, A.G. (1985). *Atlas for maxillo-facial pantomographic interpretation.* Quintessence Publications.

Langland, O.E., Langlais, E., and Morris, C. (1982). *Principles and practice of panoramic radiology.* W.B. Saunders, Philadelphia.

Wall, B.F., Fisher, E.S., Paynter, R., Hudson, A., and Bird, P. (1979). Doses to patients from pantomography — a conventional dental radiograph. *British Journal of Radiology,* **52,** 727–34.

Waites, E. (1996). *Essentials of dental radiography and radiology* (2nd edn). Churchill Livingstone, Edinburgh.

Goaz, P.W. and White, S.C. (1994). *Oral radiology principles and interpretation* (3rd edn) Mosby, St. Louis.

12 Dental radiography for children

The application of radiography in paediatric dentistry does not involve any special techniques. Standard techniques are used within the limitations of the patient's co-operation and this often depends on how well prepared the child is by the dentist, parent, or radiographer. As with all aspects of dentistry, there is an issue of consent with children — as indeed there is with adults. Children's wishes should be included in decisions involving their health care, and taking radiographs is part of their treatment.

The main points to remember are that speed is important and that lead protection should be used for both parent and child. Although lead aprons have been declared unnecessary, it gains the parent's trust in the operator in caring for the child.

12.1   FROM BIRTH TO 3 YEARS OLD

If radiography is necessary to confirm diagnosis in this age group, the usual practical means of X-raying the patient are:

- oblique lateral techniques
- mid-line oblique occlusal radiographs

Dental panoramic tomography should not be ruled out, especially in a co-operative 2–3-year-old. Some panoramic machines have the patient seated facing the operator, which helps to encourage the child to keep still (Fig. 12.1).

Radiographs are taken to demonstrate:

- caries and the extent of dental disease
- trauma, especially in the incisors
- the presence of teeth.

The oblique lateral projection can be undertaken with the patient lying prone on a horizontal surface, and the parent — suitably protected with a lead apron — holding the child:

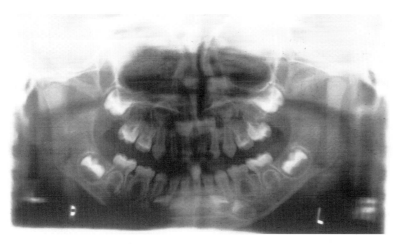

Fig. 12.1 Dental panoramic tomogram of a 3-year-old.

1. It is essential that the arms should be firmly held away from the head.

2. The head should be rotated as for the canine position.

3. The mandible should be well extended from the spine.

4. If the ramus is to be demonstrated, the head is placed in the lateral position, the mandible extended, and a good angle of separation given (Fig. 12.2).

5. The exposure factors should be adapted to reduce the time factor to a minimum.

An alternative method is with the child seated on the parent's lap; leaning up against the cassette which is rested on the parent's chest. Lead protection should be used on both child and parent.

Key points

1. Dental panoramic tomography may be possible
2. If dental panoramic tomography is not feasible, then oblique laterals are done
3. Mid-line oblique occlusals will demonstrate the anterior regions
4. Sedation may be necessary if child is distressed

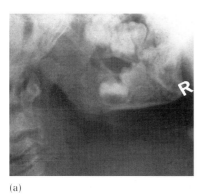
(a)

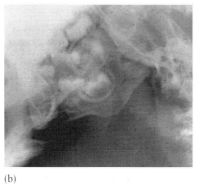
(b)

Fig. 12.2 Oblique laterals of the rami of the mandible showing hypoplasia of the left ramus and condyle in a child of 18 months.

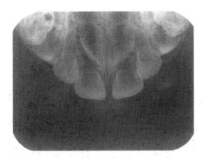

Fig. 12.3   Upper mid-line occlusal of a 9-month-old infant.

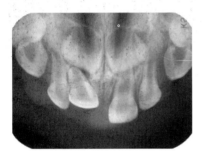

Fig. 12.4   Upper mid-line oblique occlusal on an 18-month-old child, taken to show position of the anterior teeth after trauma.

Mid-line oblique occlusal techniques may be attempted, if essential, but speed is vital. The film can be attached to a wooden spatula with tape, and the parent can stand or sit behind the child, holding the mouth closed (Figs 12.3 and 12.4).

Sometimes, the child is so distressed or unable to co-operate that sedation may be necessary to obtain any radiographs.

12.2   FROM 3 TO 6 YEARS OLD

By this age, most children will co-operate if the operator has patience and carefully explains the procedure to be undertaken. If any difficulty in co-operation is found, it is usually due to fear, so, to go through the motions of a simple mid-line oblique occlusal procedure — with the apparatus switched off — may reassure the child.

Radiographs are taken to demonstrate:

- caries and the extent of dental disease
- trauma, especially to the incisors
- developmental abnormalities
- the presence of teeth.

Dental panoramic tomography (see Chapter 11) can be undertaken with co-operative children of this age group. To help the patient keep still, it is helpful to keep their attention by a continual commentary of events (see Fig. 12.1) (Fig. 12.5). If a suitable dental panoramic tomography machine is unavailable, then oblique laterals (are performed with mid-line oblique occlusals to cover the anterior regions of the maxilla and mandible (Figs 12.6–12.9). Or, if the child will allow, bitewings can be obtained instead of obliques (Fig. 12.10).

Fig. 12.5   Panelipse tomogram of a child about 4 years old, taken to demonstrate the presence of the developing adult dentition and the state of the deciduous dentition.

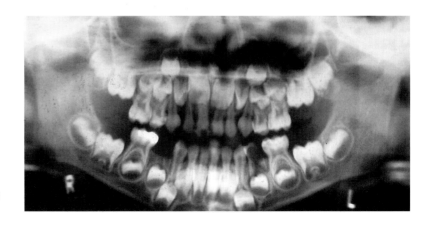

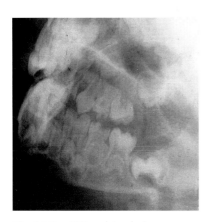

Fig. 12.6   Oblique lateral of a
3-year-old child, showing caries. This
view was taken when a bitewing film
proved impossible.

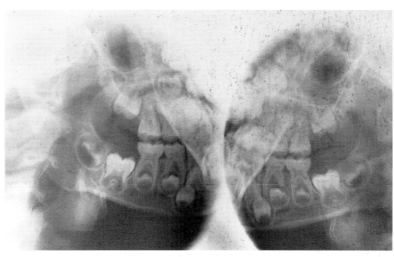

Fig. 12.7   Oblique laterals taken on one film to demonstrate position and number of
erupting teeth on a 3-year-old child.

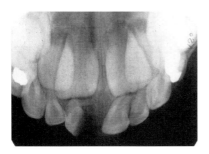

Fig. 12.8   Upper mid-line oblique of a
3-year-old child showing dilacerated
right A.

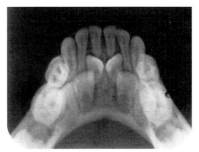

Fig. 12.9   Lower mid-line oblique
occlusal of a 3-year-old child.

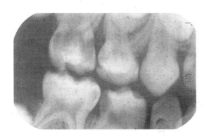
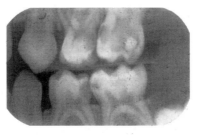

Fig. 12.10   Bitewings, using 2.2 × 3.5 cm films for a 5-year-old child.

12.2.1   Bitewing views

1. Using the 2.2 × 3.5 cm film, with the long axis parallel with the crowns and a biting tab, bitewings should be possible.
2. It is of vital importance not to cause discomfort to the child, so the anterior corners of the film must be carefully moulded.
3. It is not necessary for the film to achieve contact with the crowns, so the film should be placed with the anterior edge alongside the incisors, about 3–5 mm away from the deciduous canine and premolar teeth.
4. Apart from gaining the patient's co-operation, bitewings will, in fact, make it easier to demonstrate the interdental spaces.
5. The X-ray beam can be directed through the spaces and at 90° to the film.

12.2.2   Oblique laterals

If the patient is unable to co-operative due to a brisk gag reflex, or the position and presence of a second dentition are required, then oblique laterals should be undertaken (see Fig. 12.7)

1. This technique may be managed with the patient's head in the horizontal plane, either on the dental chair, or sitting and leaning over on to a horizontal surface.
2. Another position which can be useful is to have the child standing and leaning over the dental chair, using this as the horizontal surface.
3. The important factor is to find a method whereby the position of the head can be easily achieved, immobilized satisfactorily, and the radiograph swiftly completed.
4. Depending upon the information required, the head is positioned as for the premolar or canine region of the mandible and maxilla.
5. Both sides may be demonstrated on an 18 × 24 cm film.

Bisecting angle periapical technique can often be successfully undertaken using 2.2 × 3.5 cm film, in the deciduous molar regions. Film holders are usually easier for the patient, otherwise the child may hold the film. If this technique is impossible, oblique occlusal projections, with the standard size dental film, can nearly always be achieved.

In this age group, it is recommended that the radiographic examination should be undertaken before the child becomes too tired — in other words, near the beginning of the dental appointment and treatment.

Key points

1. Dental panoramic tomography should be achievable with care
2. If not, then oblique laterals and occlusals can be done
3. Bitewings may be possible
4. Again, if not, then oblique laterals can be done
5. Periapicals are feasible by bisecting angle technique

12.3   FROM 6 TO 12 YEARS OLD

In this age group, the co-operation is variable, mainly due to a good or bad previous experience — if the child has had an unfortunate earlier experience with X-rays, it may be more difficult to gain his or her confidence. However, at this age, it is easier to explain the procedure about to be undertaken — though in younger children, a mock film may be helpful.

Radiographs are taken to demonstrate:

- caries and the extent of dental disease
- trauma, especially to the incisors
- developmental abnormalities
- the presence of teeth.

The normal standard techniques can be employed for intra-orals using whichever size film is appropriate to the size of the mouth. Remember that to keep the film flat is all important, and it is always better to increase the angle between the film and tooth, and compensate by an increased X-ray beam angle — particularly where the mixed dentition is to be demonstrated.

Upper molar teeth are particularly difficult to radiograph as the adult film must be used to cover the 'adult' tooth, and the child finds this uncomfortable, struggling to keep the film flat and behind the tooth. Often, the angulation needs to be increased to 40° to the occlusal plane.

Speed is all important, so use the external centring point. Bitewings are reasonably easy to obtain (Fig. 12.11) and extra-oral views can be taken, as appropriate.

Key points
1. Dental panoramic tomography is easily achievable
2. Intra-oral may be possible with care
3. Bitewings are possible

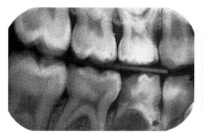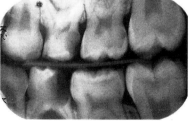

Fig. 12.11   Bitewings, using 2.2 × 3.5 cm films for a 7-year-old child.

REFERENCES AND FURTHER READING

Buckle, C.M.E. (1976). Immobilisation of the patient in paediatric radiography. *Radiography,* **XLII**, 196.

Kennedy, D. (1986). Paediatric operative dentistry (3rd edn) P.S.G. Wright, Bristol.

13 Sialography — radiography of the salivary glands and ducts

The major salivary glands — the parotid and submandibular — are paired and situated bilaterally. As soft tissue structures, they will not be demonstrated radiographically unless a radiopaque medium has been injected into their duct systems. This procedure is called 'sialography.'

The indications for this procedure are to demonstrate:

(1) stones in the salivary ducts

(2) duct strictures

(3) pathological processes within the gland, or outside the gland but compressing it.

- Where acute infection is present, sialography is contra-indicated.
- It is usual to take 'plain' films before considering this examination to demonstrate the presence of calcified stones in the duct or gland substance. (Some stones or calculi will be insufficiently calcified to be demonstrated on the plain films.)

13.1 DEMONSTRATION OF STONES IN THE DUCT

13.1.1 Parotid gland

Intra-oral view

1. A periapical film is placed in the vestibule of the mouth, adjacent to the upper molar region.
   - X-ray beam is directed 10° downwards into the film.
   - soft tissue exposure factors (Fig. 13.1(a)).
2. An occlusal film is placed into the mouth and pushed well out into the cheek on the affected side. The X-ray beam is directed downwards at 65° along the line of the duct from the gland and tangentially to the zygomatic arch (Fig. 13.1(c)).

Postero-anterior-tangential view

- The patient sits facing the film. (The use of a grid is optional.)
- OM line is parallel to the floor.

Key points

Radiographic views taken for stones in parotid duct
1. Intra-oral
   — in vestibule of mouth
      — upper molar region
   — tangential occlusal
2. Extra-oral
   — tangential posterior-anterior

- Sagittal plane is vertical.
- Affected side is at the centre of the film
- Mandible is rotated 5–10° away from the film.
- X-ray beam is parallel to the floor, tangentially along the line of the ramus.
- Centring point is midway between the condylar head and the angle of the ramus.
- Anode–film distance is 90 cm.
- Soft tissue exposure factors.

(Fig. 13.1(b))

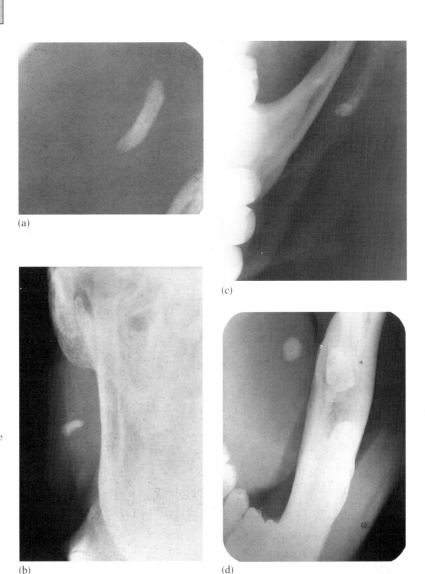

Fig. 13.1 (a) Lateral soft tissue film placed in the vestibule of the mouth in the upper molar region, demonstrating parotid calculus in the duct. (b) The same calculus, freed from superimposition of the ramus by rotation of the head. (c) Tangential view of the posterior part of the parotid duct. The beam is directed 65° from behind, downwards along the zygomatic arch. A stone is demonstrated. (d) Lower occlusal for the posterior part of the submandibular duct, showing a calculus. Reduced exposure for soft tissues.

(a)

(b)

(c)

(d)

13.1.2   Submandibular gland

Intra-oral projections

1. True occlusal view for the floor of the mouth; place the film in the mouth with its long axis along the line of the affected duct. For a
    *   Centring point is 3 cm below symphysis menti and 1 cm over the affected side.
    *   X-ray beam is 90° to the film.
    *   Anode–film distance is 30 cm.
    *   Soft tissue exposure factors.

2. For a lower lateral occlusal place the film longitudinally in the mouth, as far back as possible on the affected side. Tilt the head back, to place the occlusal plane near the vertical, and then rotate the head away from the affected side.
    *   Centring point is 1 cm inside the angle of the mandible
    *   X-ray beam is upwards at 110° to the film, along the line of the ramus of the mandible.
    *   Anode–film distance is 30 cm.
    *   Soft tissue exposure factors.

(Fig. 13.1(d))

Extra-oral views
Unless the stone is large and well calcified, it is often difficult to demonstrate in extra-oral views. Dental panoramic tomography and oblique lateral projections of the mandible may show a stone coincidentally (Fig. 13.2). Extra-glandular calcifications, such as phleboliths and tonsilloliths, will also be seen on these views (see Fig. 9.15, p. 159).

> **Key points**
>
> *Radiographic views taken for stones in submandibular duct*
> 1. True occlusal
> 2. Lower lateral occlusal
> 3. Extra-oral dental panoramic tomography or oblique lateral — Not routine, coincidental evidence of stones

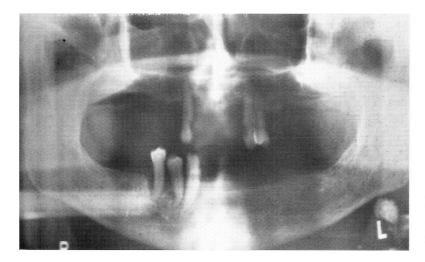

Fig. 13.2   Panelipse dental panoramic tomogram which showed, incidentally, a calcified body in the left submandibular region which was subsequently shown to be a calculus in the duct.

13.2 SIALOGRAPHY: CONTRAST MEDIA

- Oil-based, (ionic) for example, Lipiodol Ultra fluid, pantopaque.
- Water-based (ionic), for example, Hypaque Urografin, Conray (non-ionic), for example, Niopam, Ultravist.

There are indications for both types of contrast media with their consequent different modes of injection. Oil-based contrasts, however, are little used nowadays. They seem to cause the patient more discomfort, and are more likely to present granulomatous formation.

1. The oil-based media outline the gland and the duct system — any obstruction or pathological process is seen very clearly.
2. On the other hand, the water-based media are rapidly expelled and can be used more easily to judge the activity of the gland in terms of rapidity of emptying. Their opacity is not as intense as the oil-based media.
3. However, both methods depend very much on the skill of the operator, both at performing and interpreting the sialogram.

Many of the contrast media are iodine based, so these are contra-indicated when the patient is allergic to iodine.

13.2.1   Oil-based media

Hand injection methods with a cannula are sometimes used. It is possible to use a syringe, with a combination of a blunt needle and polyvinyl catheter (Manaskil 1978) which are removed before the taking of the radiographs, but extreme speed is essential before the radiopaque medium has been expelled. This method is used mainly for the parotid gland. Alternatively, special fine catheters are now available which may be used. The advantage of these is that they can be retained after the injection and held by the patient or 'strapped' to the patient's forehead. This allows the ultra-fluid form of this radiopaque medium which is much easier to inject, to be used.

The amount of radiopaque medium injected is about 1 ml for the parotid gland and 0.5 ml for the submandibular gland. The actual amount is monitored by the discomfort of the patients, but if not enough has been injected at the first attempt, more may be added.

13.2.2 Water-based media

These media are used with the hydrostatic method because they have similar characteristics to saliva and are introduced into the duct at a constant pressure just greater than the pressure of the salivary gland. A catheter is placed into the duct, which is connected to a glass syringe attached to a drip stand or the X-ray tube casing. A tap is interposed to allow the flow to be controlled. The radiographs are taken at the onset of pain, in the filling stage.

This technique — described by Mason and Chisholm (1975) — has been further developed with continuous infusion and pressure monitoring, and described by Ferguson, Evans, and Mason (1977). They advocate its use to prevent overfilling.

13.3   RADIOGRAPHIC PROCEDURE

The patient may be erect or supine for either method, but it is more usual for the hand injection to be undertaken with the patient in the sitting position, and for the patient to be supine for the hydrostatic method. The described radiographic views may be taken in either position.

When the needle method is used, the radiographs should be taken as quickly as possible, starting with the views for the gland. If possible, position the patient before the needle is removed from the duct.

Two views, at right angles, are necessary for satisfactory interpretation of sialography.

13.3.1   Parotid sialograms

1. True lateral
The patient is positioned with the head in the true lateral, and the mandible fully extended.

- Centring point is 2 cm behind the angle of the mandible.
- Normal exposure factors (Fig. 13.3a)

2. Postero-anterior (PA)
The patient is placed in the true PA position, with the affected gland in the centre of the film.

- Centring point is 2 cm above the angle of the mandible.
- Exposure factors are decreased by 30%, Fig. 13.3(b).

Key points

Radiographic views taken for parotid sialogram
Extra-oral views

— true lateral
— posterio-anterior
— 30° occipitomental

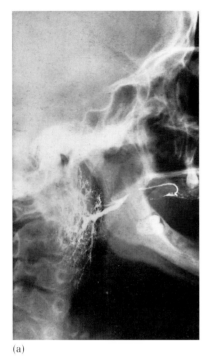

(a)

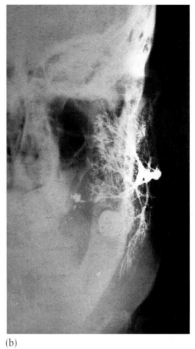

(b)

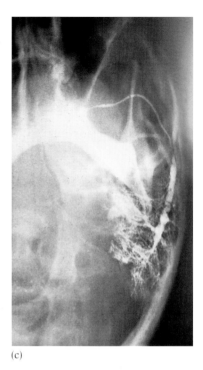

(c)

Fig. 13.3   (a) Lateral view; (b) poster-anterior view; (c) 30° occipitomental view —
this projection demonstrates stenosis in the main duct.

3. 30° Occipitomental (OM)
The patient is placed in the true OM position, with the X-ray beam
angled towards the orbital-meatal line at 30°. The affected gland is in
the centre of the film.

- Centring point is 2.5 cm above the external occipital protuberance, to the affected side.
- Exposure factors are increased by 20%, Fig. 13.3(c).

This projection demonstrates the parotid duct, as well as the gland. It
is usually undertaken with a skull unit, which may not be necessary
when digital techniques are employed.

13.3.2   Submandibular sialograms

1. Lateral
The patient is placed with the head in the true lateral position, and
the mandible fully extended from the spine. The film should be parallel to the sagittal plane and placed in a film holder, with or without a
grid. Alternatively, the patient may hold the film.

Key points

*Radiographic views taken for
submandibular sialogram*
extra-oral views
  true lateral
  rotational panoramic
  intra oral tomography
  lateral oblique occlusal
  true occlusal

- Centring point is 2.5 cm below the angle of the mandible.
- X-ray beam is 5° to the film and sagittal plane.
- Exposure factors are decreased by 30%.

(Fig. 13.4(a))

2. Lower lateral oblique occlusal
Care must be taken to insert the film into the mouth so that the gland and duct are centrally placed (Fig. 13.4(b)).

3. True occlusal
Both these intra-oral views are taken as for the 'plain' films, but with normal exposure factors (Fig. 13.4(c)).

4. Dental panoramic tomography (see Chapter 11)
This projection may be used instead of the lateral or oblique lateral views, in either parotid or submandibular sialography. It is most useful when a catheter method is employed and the opaque medium remains within the gland. To bring the gland into the focal trough, the head should be brought forwards and the sagittal plane may be tilted about 10° away from the affected side — but this is difficult to judge precisely (Fig. 13.5).

In the hydrostatic method, the flow of contrasting agent is stopped by closing the tap between each exposure to prevent unnecessary distension of the gland.

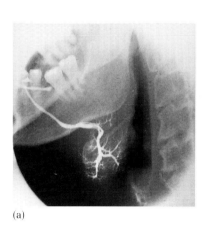
(a)

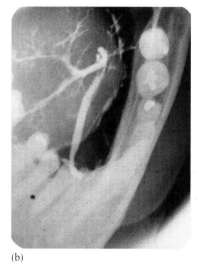
(b)

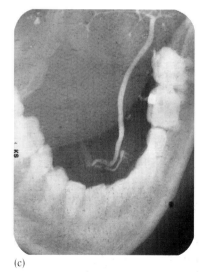
(c)

Fig. 13.4 (a) Lateral projection with 5° upwards angulation. A small amount of swallowed contrast medium accidentally outlines the pharynx. (b) Lateral occlusal with oblique projection to demonstrate the submandibular gland. (c) On a different patient, a true occlusal demonstrates the course of the submandibular duct. Unusually, the sublingual gland has also been filled by the contrast medium, due to an exit duct shared with the submandibular gland.

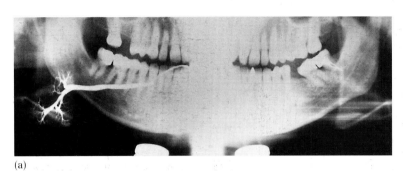

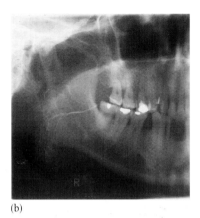

(a)   (b)

Fig. 13.5   (a) Panorex dental panoramic tomograph to demonstrate right submandibular sialogram. (b) Orthophos radiograph of the right submandibular gland. This demonstrates the evolvement of dental panoramic tomography, enabling only the specific area of interest to be radiographed and, thus, reducing the radiation exposure.

With this method, when occlusal films may not be possible, a rotated oblique lateral is taken to demonstrate the more anterior portion of the mandibular duct.

- In both parotid and submandibular sialography, these radiographs may be repeated at 10–60 minute intervals, to monitor emptying time.
- This may be particularly useful when a catheter is retained in position during the original series, preventing the natural flow of saliva with the expulsion of the contrast medium.

13.4   NEW IMAGING TECHNIQUES

The new imaging techniques are especially useful for investigating the soft tissue structure of salivary glands and for associated pathology.

13.4.1   Digital fluoroscopy

In many medical departments, sialography is carried out under direct digital fluoroscopy. The salivary gland is injected with contrast under direct visualization (*real time imaging*). This helps to eliminate overfilling of the gland, and underfilling due to lack of patient tolerance and artifacts produced by air bubbles.

Another advantage of digital fluoroscopy is that the radiologist can see the duct and gland as the contrast medium is injected, and can adjust the patient's position to demonstrate any abnormality.

It is also possible, as in direct dental digital imaging (see Ch. 7) to enhance the image.

It is important, as the radiation dosage is considerably reduced, to resist the temptation to take even more films (Fig. 13.6).

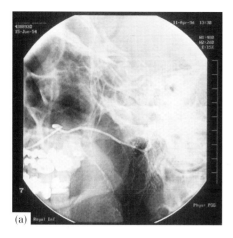 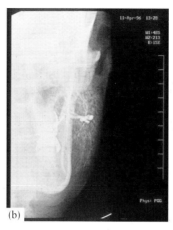

Fig. 13.6 Normal Parotid sialogram investigated with digital fluoroscopy: (a) rotated postero-anterior projection; (b) lateral projection.

13.4.2 Digital subtraction

This involves the use of an image, prior to the introduction of contrast, which functions as a mask to be electronically subtracted from subsequent images, after contrast has been given.

- The subtracted image only contains that information from the second image that differs from the first.
- This technique further enhances visualization of structures already contrast enhanced, by the elimination of background anatomy from the image.
- It is imperative when using this technique, that the patient remains completely still — any movement will distort the mask image and lead to subtraction artifact (Figs 13.7 and 13.8).

13.4.3 Radionuclide imaging

This is primarily used to assess the function of salivary glands and is of particular value in patients for whom cannulisation is a problem. A radio-isotope scan can be performed with an iv injection of a radio-nuclide (200mbq -99m pertechnetate). Normal salivary and sub-mandibular glands show up as paired areas of increased activity darkening on the digital image (Fig. 13.9). The investigation is usually over a 25 min period taking 1 frame/min on analogue images and 1 frame/30 sec on computer for time-activity graphs. After about 10 min diluted citric acid is given through a straw-sialogogue to observe the activity of the glands. Activity curves normally rise initially and then fall steeply after the sialogogue (Figs 13.10 and 13.11).

13.4.4 Ultrasound

Ultrasound is particularly helpful in the investigation of soft tissue masses. The normal parotid and submandibular glands are readily

Key points

Techniques now available within specialised hospital units
- Digital Imaging — real time
Contrast injected during imaging so helps to prevent over- or underfilling
Patient's position can be adjusted to demonstrate abnormality
Radiation dosage reduced
- Digital Subtraction
Eliminates background anatomy
- Radionuclide Imaging
Function of glands
Contrast medium — intravenous injection of radio-nuclide

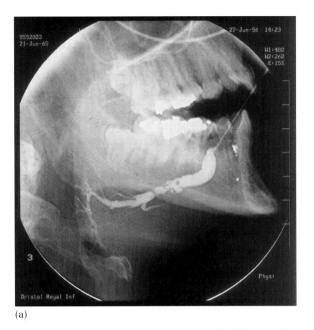

(a)

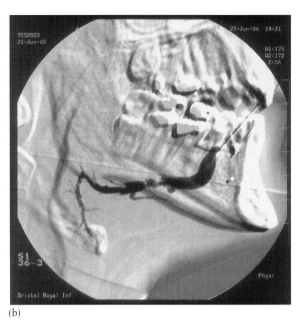

(b)

Fig. 13.7 Submandibular sialogram with a digitized image receptor: (a) lateral projection and (b) same view with subtraction, demonstrating a dilated submandibular duct with calculus, stenosis, and diverticulosis.

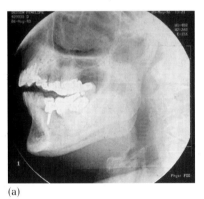

(a)

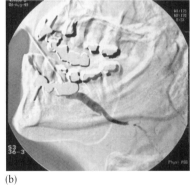

(b)

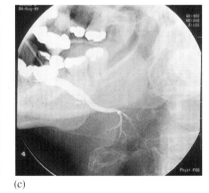

(c)

Fig. 13.8 Left submandibular sialogram carried out with digital fluoroscopy and subtraction: (a) the pre-injection lateral oblique view; (b) the post-injection subtracted view; (c) the directly digitized view. The left duct is dilated and there is a radiolucent stone within the dilated duct. Note the sublingual gland is also visualized.

identified with ultrasound but, as access to the sublingual glands is difficult, is rarely of value. A high-frequency transducer allows excellent resolution of the glands and, indeed, almost 100 per cent of masses may be identified, including those that are impalpable clinically.

Coupling gel is applied to the skin and the glands may be imaged in longitudinal transverse and oblique planes.

Parotid gland

1. The normal parotid gland has indistinct margins, with the retropharyngeal portion being difficult to visualize. Overall, the echo texture is homogeneous and slightly brighter than the surrounding muscles.

2. The normal duct may occasionally be visualized as a closely applied pair of echogenic lines.

3. The infected gland will be tender, enlarged, and relatively echo-poor.

4. Dilatation of the duct may be visible, together with intra-ductal calculi.

5. Ultrasound allows the visualization of non-radiopaque calculi.

Submandibular gland

1. The submandibular glands may be identified by their triangular shape. The echo texture is similar to that of the parotid gland.

2. Very occasionally, the duct may visualized.

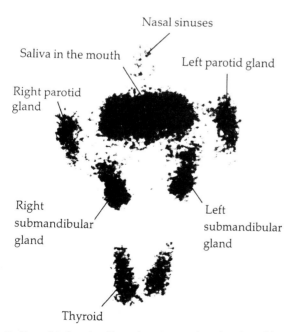

Fig. 13.9 Radionuclide Imaging Normal anatomy—Anterior view of face and neck demonstrating the parotid and submandibular salivary glands. The thyroid is included as well as saliva in the mouth.

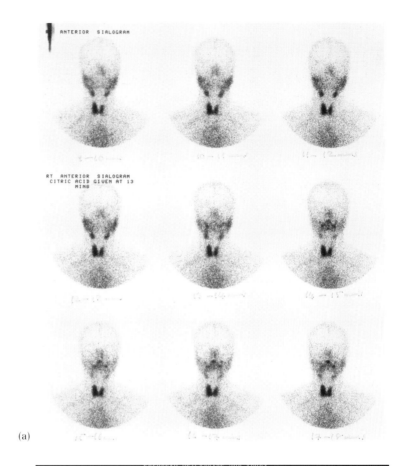

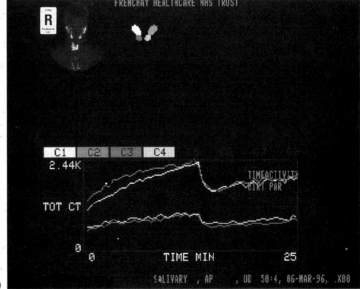

Fig. 13.10 Radionuclide Imaging (a) Computerised scan during the 9–18 minute period of the 25 minute investigation; (b) The activity curve showing the immediate fall after the citric acid was given 13 minutes. This demonstrates normal function of the glands.

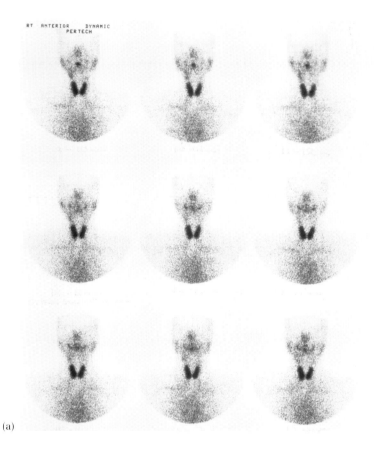

(a)

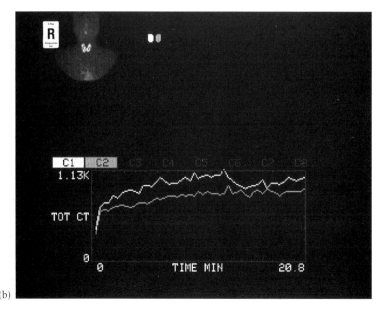

(b)

Fig. 13.11 (a) Similar investigation on patient showing less uptake of the radionuclide (less darkening) of the left submandibular gland; (b) The activity curve does not rise or fall very much demonstrating a poor function and obstructed drainage.

Key points

Ultra-sound
electronic image displayed from
high frequency sound-beam
demonstrates—soft tissue
— inflammation
— tumours

This technique has the great advantage of not involving the use of X-rays, and is a very useful tool in the investigation of salivary glands.

1. Ultrasound is of particular value for suspected inflammation and tumours.

2. The technique provides a good method to guide percutaneous aspiration and consequent drainage of abscesses within the salivary glands, characterized by an irregular outline, with an echo-poor fluid centre which may or not contain debris. spiration of an abscess under ultrasound control is generally a straight-forward procedure.

3. Patients with a palpable mass can be investigated by ultrasound to demonstrate. differences between intra-and extra-glandular lesions, and to help in predicting whether these are benign or malignant.

    • Benign masses, such as adenomas, are generally echo-poor with well-defined margins.
    • Malignant conditions, however, are generally ill defined, and are often lobulated with a heterogeneous echo texture (Fig. 13.12).

Other specialized techniques — computerized tomography (CT) and magnetic resonance imaging (MRI) — are also especially useful in locating and diagnosing benign and malignant tumours. (Fig. 13.13) (see Chapter 14.)

With the new imaging techniques evolving, there may come a time when Sialography will not be the investigation of choice. Though

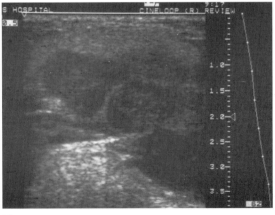

(a)

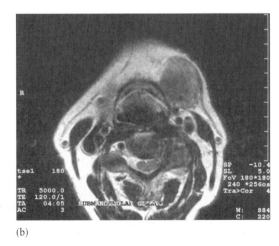

(b)

Fig. 13.12   (a) Ultra sound image demonstrating a submandibular malignant tumour; (b) MRI axial view of the same patient.

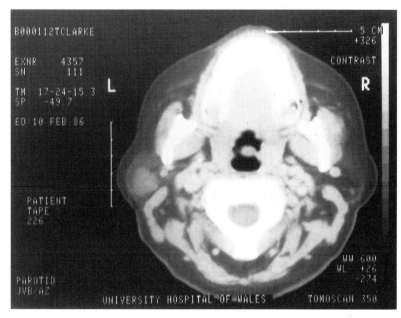

Fig. 13.13   C.T Shows a well circumscribed lesion of increased density in the left parotid gland consistent with a benign tumour.

outside the province of the general practitioner, the techniques are very relevant within the dento-maxillofacial field.

REFERENCES AND FURTHER READING

Kurabayashi, T. *et al.* (1997). Differential diagnosis of tumours of the minor salivary glands of the palate by CT. *Journal of the International Association of Dentomaxillofacial Radiology,* **26** 21.

Croce, F., Derchi, E., and Soibiati, I. *Salivary glands. Clinical Ultrasound, volume 2* (ed. Miere, Cosgrove, Dewbury, and Wilde). Churchill Livingstone, Edinburgh.

Waites, E. (1996) *Essentials of dental radiography and radiology* (2nd edn). Churchill Livingstone, Edinburgh.

Ferguson, M.M., Evans, A., and Mason, W.N. (1997). *International Journal of Oral Surgery,* **6**, 84–9.

Morse, M.H. (1995). Salivary gland imaging. In *Colour atlas and text* (ed. J.E. Deburgh–Norman and M.M. Gurk). Mosby-White.

Manaskil, G.B. (1978). *Clinical sialography.* Thoman, Illinois.

Mason, D.K. and Chisholm, D.M. (1975). *Salivary glands in health and disease.* W.B. Saunders, Philadelphia.

Pappas, G.C. and Wallace, W.R. (1980). *Panoramic sialography.* (Table demonstration at the 5th International Congress of Dento-Maxillo-Facial Radiology, 1980.)

Seward, G.R. (1981). The salivary glands. In *Bailey and Love's short practice of surgery.* (ed. A.J. Harding-Rains and H.D. Richie), pp. 583–97. H.K. Lewis, London.

Whyte, A.M. and Byrne, J.D. (1987). A comparison of computer tomography and ultrasound in the assessment of parotid masses. *Clinical Pathology,* **38**, 339–43.

Luyk, N.H., Doyle, T., and Ferguson, M.M. (1992). Recent trends in imaging salivary glands. *Journal for the International Association of Dento-maxillofacial Radiology,* **20**, No. 1, Butterworth-Heinemann.

Lewis, M.A.O., Lamey, P.J., Straney, R., and Mason, W.N. (1992). Clinical application of computerised continuous-infusion pressure monitored sialography. *Journal for the International Association of Dento-maxillofacial Radiology,* **20**. No. 2, Butterworth-Heinemann.

Kurabayashi, T. *et al.* (1992). Radiographic quality and patient discomfort: comparison of iohexol with iothalamate. *Journal for the International Association of Dento-maxillofacial* Radiology, **20**, No. 2, Butterworth-Heinemann.

14   Specialized techniques

In conventional radiography, the direction of the X-ray beam does not change during exposure, and only those boundaries of structures within the subject which have surfaces that are parallel to the beam are recorded on the film.

14.1   TOMOGRAPHY

Tomography is a form of radiography where it is possible to focus on one layer or section of a 'body' (hence its name; *tome* is Greek for section or cut).

The principle of tomography is that the X-ray source and the film move in opposite directions across the object, with a constant ratio between their velocities about a pivot point. In this system, the rays falling upon a fixed point on the film throughout the exposure will have a point of intersection that is stationary in relation to the object during exposure. When these conditions are met, each point lying upon a particular plane within the object will be projected exactly on the film during the entire motion. This is called the focal plane or cut (Fig. 14.1). The larger the arc of movement or the exposure angle, the more precisely it is possible to focus to a narrow plane. Variation in the exposure angle can produce variations in the depth of the focal cut.

The equipment used for this method of imaging is specialized for example Scanora, Tomax, or adapted X-ray equipment in a medical imaging department (Fig. 14.2). There are a range of movements which can be performed on these machines, the simplest being linear and the most complicated, hypocycloidal. It is possible to take multi-layer tomography on the adapted X-ray equipment, by placing films in a special cassette sandwiched between layers of polystyrene. Each film will have a constant relationship — that is, a constant velocity ratio — with a different layer or tomography cut within the object, during the exposure travel (Figs 14.3 and 14.4).

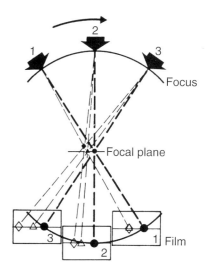

Fig. 14.1   Diagram showing the principle of tomography. ● is the centre of the focal plane and its image maintains its position on the film during the opposing arc-like movement of the X-ray tube and the film. Point △ on the focal plane maintains its relevant position on the film to ●. Point ◇, a point in a different plane, is purposely blurred due to its changing relationship to the film (after Ando 1971).

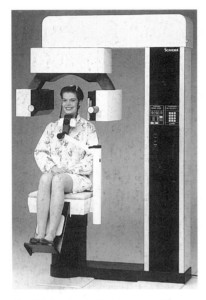

Fig. 14.2   Specialized tomographic equipment.

Applications

- Assessment of the temporomandibular joint (TMJ) both anterio-posterior (AP) and lateral
- Assessment of the rami of the jaw, AP and lateral
- Assessment of the height and width of the jaw for implants
- Assessment of the facial bones for fractures after trauma
- Assessment of the orbit for blow out fractures

Advantages

- Easy to perform
- Relatively cheap
- No appointment is necessary
- The dose is comparatively low compared to that of computerized tomography (CT)

Disadvantages

- Specialized equipment is required
- Lack of detail on films compared to conventional radiography
- The patient must remain in the same position for some time

It is worth nothing that this principle of tomography has been developed extensively and is behind much of the modern imaging technology, for example, CT scanning, magnetic resonance imaging (MRI), and positron emission, where it may be applied in the axial and sagittal or median planes.

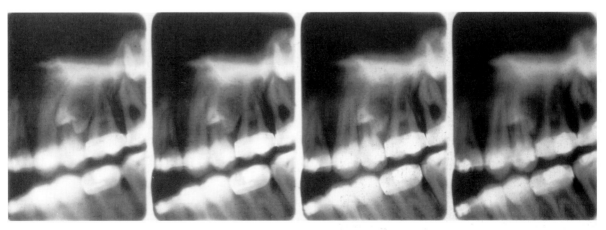

Fig. 14.3   Tangential tomographic images using specialized tomographic equipment which ensures a constant magnification. These images show the relationship of an impacted upper premolar to the other teeth.

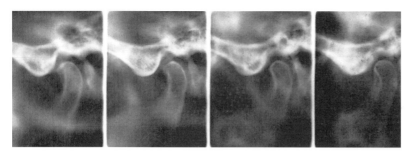

Fig. 14.4   Lateral tomograms of the TMJ.

Key points

- Tomography is used to demonstrate thin planes within the body
- This is achieved by moving the X-ray tube and the film about a pivot point
- It requires specialised equipment
- It is used to demonstrate areas not easily seen on conventional radiograpy
- C.T. utilises the same principal as tomography with the use of a computer
- It produces sectional images usually in the axial plane
- The images can be reconstructed in any plane
- Demonstrates small differences in tissue density

14.2   COMPUTERIZED TOMOGRAPHY (CT)

CT scanning consists of an X-ray tube attached to an array of detectors to produce sectional images, usually in the axial plane. The detectors measure the amount of radiation emanating from the patient and, with the use of a computer, convert the information into a visual image.

In the last few years, the technology has improved to produce scanners in which the X-ray tube rotates within a stationary ring of detectors. This means that the time of each scan is reduced. The patient moves through the machine and multiple contiguous scans are imaged, which can then be viewed in the axial, coronal, or sagittal plane.

Since the resolution is high contrast, and the technique can demonstrate small differences in tissue density, CT is useful in the diagnosis of disease in the head and neck (Figs 14.5 and 14.6).

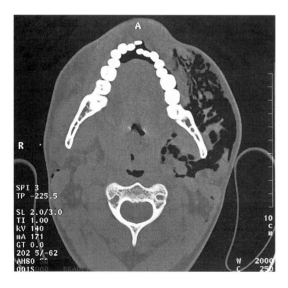

Fig. 14.5   Axial CT scan of the mandible, demonstrating air in the soft tissues as well as a displaced fracture of the anterior portion of the mandible.

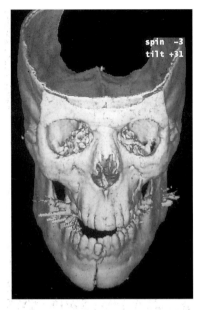

Fig. 14.6   3D reconstruction from the axial scans of Fig. 14.5, demonstrating the facial bones and mandible. Note artefact from the fillings in the teeth.

Applications

- Evaluation of the jaws prior to interosseous implants
- Investigation of intercranial disease
- Investigation of the head and neck, post trauma
- Examination of benign and malignant tumours
- Assessment of fractures of the head and neck
- Investigation of the TMJ
- Investigation of the salivary glands

Advantages

- Hard and soft tissues imaged
- Demonstrates small differences in soft tissue density
- Eliminates superimposition of structures
- Axial images produced
- Sagittal and coronal reconstructions can be obtained
- 3-D images can be obtained, with the relevant software.

Disadvantages

- Not readily available
- Expensive
- Relatively high dose of radiation
- Artefacts introduced by metal, for example fillings

14.3   MAGNETIC RESONANCE IMAGING (MRI)

Unlike the previously discussed modalities, MRI does not use X-radiation to produce images, but magnetism. The patient lies in a large magnetic field, to which the nuclei of many of the atoms in the body to align themselves. Radio-frequency pulses are applied, and the atoms change their alignment; following the radio-frequency pulse, the atoms return to their original positions. As the atoms relax back to their normal state, they emit a radio-wave signal. This signal is detected and fed into a computer which produces an image. These images can be reconstructed in any plane (Fig 14.7).

Applications

- To demonstrate soft tissue abnormalities in the salivary glands and the neck
- To demonstrate lesions in the brain and the spinal cord
- Assessment of the TMJ

Advantages

• Information can be reconstructed in any plane
• No ionizing radiation
• Soft tissue differentiation well demonstrated
• No contrast media required

Disadvantages

• Not readily available
• Scan times can be lengthy, introducing movement artefacts in the images
• Expensive
• Contra-indicated in patients with metal clips, for example aneurysm clips or cardiac pacemakers.

14.4   ULTRASOUND

Diagnostic ultrasound uses high-frequency sound, directed into the body from a transducer placed in contact with the skin, to produce images. The skin needs to be covered with a 'coupling' medium — either oil or jelly — to make good acoustic contact. As the sound travels through the body, some of it is reflected back by tissue interfaces to produce echoes which are picked up by the same transducer and converted into electrical signals which then produce a visual image (Fig. 14.8).

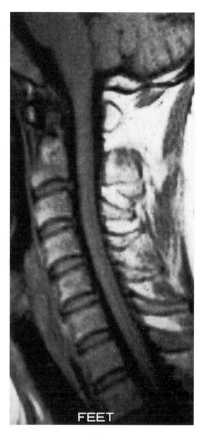

Fig. 14.7   Sagittal MRI reconstruction of the cervical portion of the spinal cord.

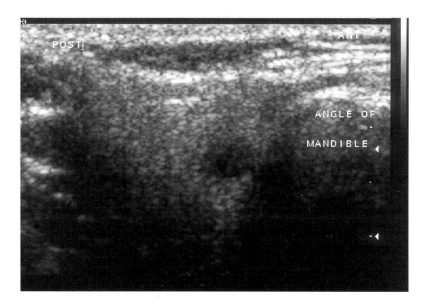

Fig. 14.8   Transverse ultrasound of a normal parotid gland demonstrating the angle of the mandible anteriorly and posteriorly the belly of diagastric and facial artery centrally.

Air, bone, and other calcified tissues absorb the ultrasound beam. However, other tissues produce distinctive echo patterns.

Applications

- Evaluation of lymph nodes in the neck
- Assessment of post-operative oedema or haematoma
- Evaluation of the thyroid, parotid, and submandibular glands (see Chapter 13)
- Assessment of carotid blood flow

Advantages

- No ionizing radiation is used, only high-frequency sound
- Easily available and relatively inexpensive
- Good soft tissue differentiation

Disadvantages

- Images can be difficult to interpret
- Limited use in the head and neck
- Ultrasound is operator dependent

14.5   RADIOISOTOPE IMAGING

Radioactive isotopes, used in diagnostic imaging, emit gamma rays as they decay which are detected by a gamma camera which then produces an image.

Gamma rays are electromagnetic radiation which are produced by the decay of the nucleus. Radioisotopes used in medical diagnosis are artificially produced and have short half lives. Radioisotope imaging depends on the isotope to be used 'tagging' on to certain substances which concentrate in certain parts of the body. Technetium 99m is the most commonly used isotope since it has a half life of only six hours and emits gamma radiation of an energy which is easily detected (Fig. 14.9).

A development of radioisotope imaging — single photon emission computerized tomography (SPECT) — is utilized to demonstrate tumour invasion of the mandible by intra-oral squamous cell carcinoma. The gamma camera moves around the patient to produce sectional images similar to CT (Fig. 14.10). This technique can also be used to ascertain the viability of bone grafts in the mandible and to demonstrate the salivary glands (see chapter 13).

Positron emission tomography (PET) is another more recent development in the field of radioisotope imaging. Use of this technique is still limited, due to high costs and the need for an on-site cyclotron to generate the positron emitting radioisotopes.

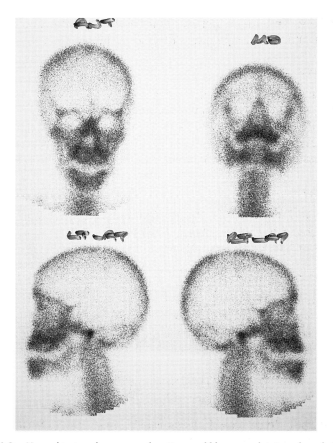

Fig. 14.9 Normal isotope bone scan of an 8-year-old boy complaining of a palpable bony swelling of the right maxilla. The patient was injected with 23g MBq Tc99m MDP, and imaged 3 hours post injection using a high-resolution collimator 128×128 matrix.

Applications

- Investigation of bone lesions
- Information on salivary gland function
- Investigation of the thyroid gland
- Assessment of TMJ growth

Advantages

- All target tissues can be imaged at the same time, for example, all salivary glands
- Function of the target tissue is measured

Disadvantages

- Relatively poor spatial resolution of the images
- Radiation dose can be relatively high

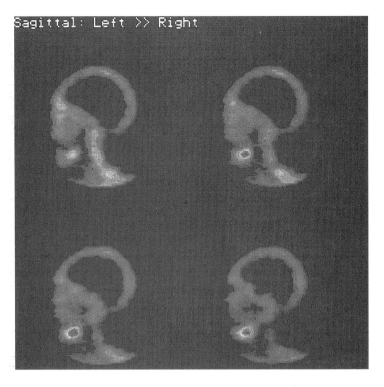

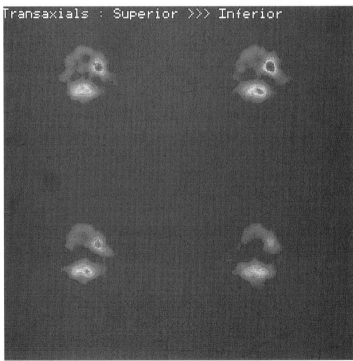

Fig. 14.10 SPECT study demonstrating abnormal uptake of tracer in the left mandible due to squamous cell carcinoma.

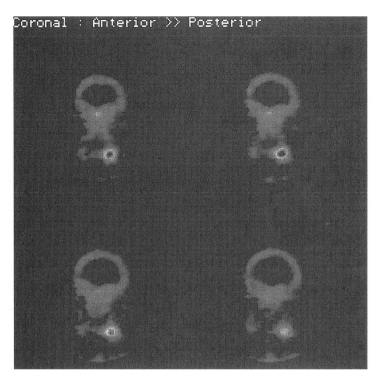

Fig. 14.10 *continued*

Key points

- MRI uses magnetism not radiation
- The images can be reconstructed in any plane
- Soft tissue is well demonstrated
- Like CT, MRI is expensive
- Ultrasound does not use radiation
- Easily available and cheap
- Operator dependant
- Radioisotopes emit gamma rays which are detected and produce images
- Function of target tissue is measured

- Investigations can take several hours
- Images are not disease specific

REFERENCES AND FURTHER READING

Armstrong, P. and Wastie, M.L. (1992). *Diagnostic imaging* (3rd edn) Blackwell Scientific Publications, Oxford.

Chan, K.W., Merick, M.V., and Mitchell, R. (1996). Bone SPECT to assess mandibular invasion by intraoral squamous cell carcinomas. *The Journal of Nuclear Medicine*, **37, No. 1**, p. 42–5.

Goaz, P.W. and White, S.C. (1994). *Oral radiology principles and interpretation* (3rd edn). Mosby, St. Louis.

Waites, E. (1996). *Essentials of dental radiography and radiology*, (3rd edn). Churchill Livingstone, Edinburgh.

15 Dental implants and radiography

The use of osseointegrated endosseous implants has made a major impact in aspects of restorative dentistry, and now forms a predictable treatment. The term 'osseointegration' has been defined by Zarb and Albrektsson as a process whereby a clinically rigid asymptomatic fixation of alloplastic materials is achieved and maintained, in bone, during functional loading.

A few years ago, implants were considered a last resort treatment when conventional, complete dentures had failed. Now, they are considered early on in treatment planning. The scope of use has also expanded to encompass tooth replacement in the partially edentulous patient.

This increase in implant use and the expansion in the variety of applications has made considerable demands on radiographic techniques. The requirements for radiography may be broadly divided into:

- pre-surgical planning
- restorative treatment
- maintenance monitoring of research trials
- diagnosis of the failing implant.

15.1   PRE-SURGICAL PLANNING

The primary object is to identify bone volume, close anatomical structures, and undiagnosed buried roots and pathology. Bone quality cannot be assessed reliably on routine radiographs because cortical thickness and the degree of trebeculation is not readily identified.

15.1.1   Parallel periapicals (see Chapter 4)

In the situation of a few missing teeth, a parallel radiograph gives considerable information with no or little distortion or magnification. The use of paralleling film holders are essential to accurately demonstrate bone height. However, there are problems associated with this technique, one of which is that only a small field is visualized, as it may be important to use paedodontic size films to achieve a true projection of the area. There is also difficulty in obtaining an undistorted film in areas of shallow palate and reduced sulcus depth (Fig. 15.1).

Advantages

- A true view of the bone height is achieved
- There is little distortion
- There is reduced or little magnification
- The technique is standardized and reproducible
- Comparatively low radiation dose
- Low cost

Disadvantages

- Special film holders are necessary
- A small field is visualized
- Difficult to achieve with a shallow palate or reduced sulcus depth
- In the above, there is no guarantee the film will be parallel to the area
- If the films are not parallel, there may be a variable magnification factor
- The paralleling devices are often uncomfortable, and the patient's co-operation is essential

15.1.2 Digital intra-oral radiography (see Chapter 7)

Digitized intra-oral images can be produced using image receptors as an alternative to conventional intra-oral film. This technique offers rapid acquisition of images, which are then viewed on a computer screen. Placement of the receptor is identical to that of an intra-oral film with the same advantages and disadvantages. An added advantage

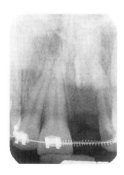 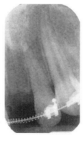

Fig. 15.1 Periapical radiograph to demonstrate bone height in upper incisor area using paralleling technique.

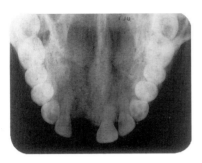

Fig. 15.2   Upper anterior occlusal radiograph.

is that the radiation dose is reduced compared to intra-oral radiography. However, the images may be manipulated to produce false positives or negatives.

15.1.3   Occlusal radiography (see Chapter 8)

This gives an idea of the spatial position of buried roots and other pathology. The cortex and cancellous bone may be viewed, but they have little bearing on implant placement as the film and X-ray beam are not parallel to the alveolar process in the upper jaw. In the lower jaw, a cross-sectional view may be obtained using a true occulsal projection, but this only shows the maximum width of bone (Fig. 15.2)

15.1.4   Lateral cephalometric radiography (see Chapter 10)

This is taken on a cephalostat, or a lateral skull view may be done on a Scanora or equivalent. The Scanora is a sophisticated piece of equipment which produces linear scanned images as well as multidirectional tomography with a constant magnification. The view can be taken with or without a stent containing metal markers.

This projection shows the proclination of the existing teeth and a good view of the maxillary sinuses. Although these views give information concerning bone availability in the premaxilla and mandibular symphysis (which is an area to be avoided for implants), their use is limited, as the median area alone is shown.

Advantages

- Easy to perform
- Easy to standardize
- Magnification is fixed
- Comparatively low radiation dose

Disadvantages

- Need the relevant equipment
- Limited use

15.1.5   Dental panoramic tomography (see Chapter 11)

These tomograms give a good overall picture, but are subject to distortion. To reduce these errors and to aid orientation, stents are often

---

Key points

- Implants have had a major impact on Restorative Dentistry
- Can be used in edentulous and partially edentulous patients
- Pre-surgical planning is to identify bone volume
- Parallel radiographs are used to measure the bone volume in the situation of a few missing teeth
- Digital imaging can be used
- Occlusal views have limited use
- Lateral cephalometric skull shows a good view of the maxilla in the median plane

used. These may be copies of a denture incorporating steel balls of known dimension, twists of wire, or vacuum-moulded splints painted with radio-opaque material. It is important to have the balls or wire as close to the implant site as possible to minimize errors in distortion calculation.

Other methods to help calculate distortion include average templates, provided by some companies, and various grids of known dimensions. The more sophisticated modern equipment, for example, Orthophos, Scanora, and Tomax, can provide an image of constant magnification. This does not reduce the distortion — that is up to the operator.

It is important to position the patient correctly and, when considering the mandible, it is important to get the lower border visible on the radiograph and to make sure there is no rotation of the head. This technique is more difficult to standardize (Fig. 15.3).

Advantages

- Shows more information
- Relatively easy to perform by the operator
- Easy for the patient
- Comparatively low radiation dose

Disadvantages

- Variable magnification depending on the type of machine used
- Some distortion can occur
- It can be difficult to position the patient correctly, especially when edentulous
- More difficult to standardize this technique

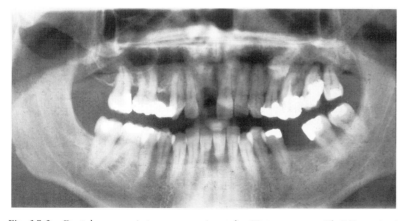

Fig. 15.3 Dental panoramic tomogram using a dentition program with 1.7 constant magnification.

15.1.6 Tomography (see Chapter 14)

This technique enables cross-sectional views of the jaws to be studied. It can help in determining available bone, bucco-lingually, and to locate, more precisely, structures like the inferior dental nerve. For these reasons, tomography is particularly useful for planning implant placement in the posterior mandible and maxilla.

The X-ray beam has to be perpendicular to the bone in the area under investigation for accurate imaging, so sophisticated equipment such as the Scanora or Tomax is essential. The magnification for individual pieces of equipment is fixed, uniform, and known. This is important for measurement taking and for standardization (Figure 15.4).

Advantages

- Accurate assessment of the bone height and volume
- Location of structures, for example, the inferior dental canal, can be identified
- Magnification is fixed
- Reasonably easy to perform
- Not too uncomfortable for the patient

Disadvantages

- Equipment not readily available
- Expensive
- Radiation dose higher than periapical films

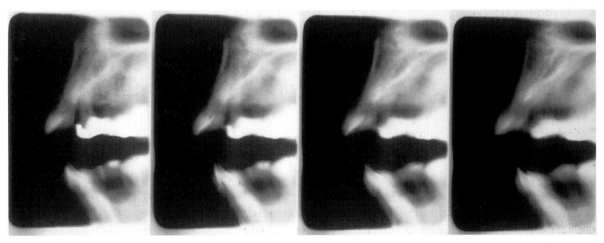

Fig. 15.4 Cross-sectional tomogram of anterior maxilla using 4 mm cuts with 1.7 constant magnification.

- The operator needs specialist training to use the equipment to its full potential
- Interpretation of the images can be confusing — the use of stents is helpful

15.1.7 Computerized tomography (see Chapter 14)

With specialist software, some CT scanners can produce images which may give precise information concerning bone availability. These would be used instead of cross-sectional tomography. Multiple 1.5 mm axial scans are performed, and the images are reformatted to produce either cross-sections of the jaw or maxilla, or axial images with a superimposed curve and panoramic views. The number of scans needed to produce these images varies, depending on the patient and the area. It is an expensive method of imaging (Fig. 15.5).

Advantages

- Displays life-size images
- Provides information on bone height and volume
- Provides bone density values
- Soft tissues can be assessed
- Relatively comfortable for the patient

Disadvantages

- Expensive
- Not readily available
- High radiation dose compared to conventional techniques
- Metallic objects cause artefact

15.2 RESTORATIVE TREATMENT

Radiographs are used to confirm osseointegration by the lack of radiolucency around the fixture (implant). Following abutment connection in some two-part systems, radiographs are often taken to confirm correct seating of the two components (Fig. 15.6). The films taken are parallel views of the fixture/abutment interface.

When the restoration is complete, radiographs are taken to obtain a baseline with which to measure any further bone loss. Reproducibility and standardization of the techniques are important, so that any changes can be accurately measured.

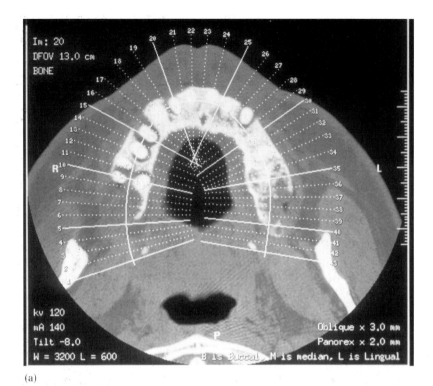

(a)

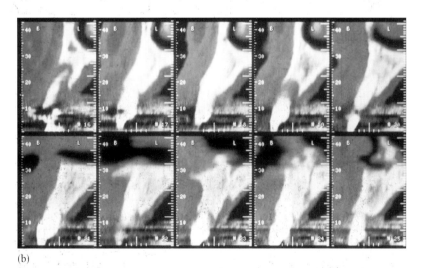

(b)

Fig. 15.5 (a) Axial CT scan of the maxilla, demonstrating computer-generated numbered cross-hatches. (b) CT cross-sectional images reconstructed from axial CT data using a selected software reformatting program. The reconstructed images contain a scale for accurate measurement. (c) CT images reformatted parallel to the alveolar ridge. There is a scale for accurate measurement.

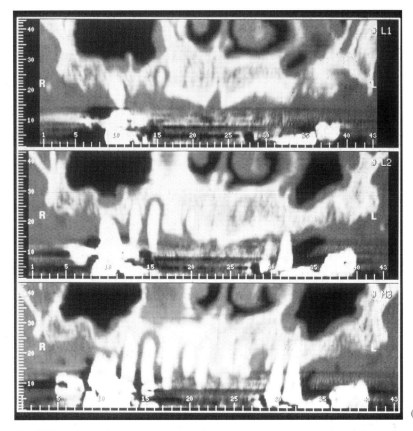

(c)

Fig. 15.5 *continued*

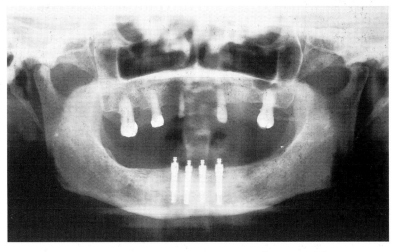

Fig. 15.6 Dental panoramic tomogram demonstrating alignment of abutments. Note the mismatch of implants in the region of 42 and 34.

Key points

- Dental Panoramic Tomography gives a good overall picture but is subject to distortion
- Tomography enables cross-sectional views of the jaw
- CT can be used but the exposure dose is very high and is expensive
- Radiographs are required to confirm osseointergration of implants
- Reproducibility and standardisation are essential for monitoring
- Failing implants are confirmed by parallel radiographs
- Co-operation of the patient is essential

The success of endosseus implants varies with implant site and length. It is expected that 2 mm of crestal bone will be lost in the first year but, thereafter, the loss should be less than 0.2 mm.

15.3 MONITORING

For research purposes, accurate reproducible films are required. Paralleling film holders are essential. Rinn film holders are often used which have the advantage of a visual guide for the X-ray beam. Precision film holders are also useful, especially with patients who have little sulcus depth. Usually, custom-made devices are constructed which attach to the implant and hold the film in a standard way (Fig. 15.7).

15.4 DIAGNOSIS OF THE FAILING IMPLANT

Confirmation of non-existent or failing integration is usually achieved by parallel view films. Intra-oral radiographs demonstrate more detail of the surrounding bone than other techniques, and paralleling is the technique of choice, as the films are comparable with previous images. Bone defects, similar to those seen in periodontal breakdown, may be seen with apical changes (Fig. 15.8).

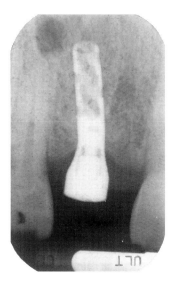

Fig. 15.7 Periapical of an implant in the upper incisor area, using paralleling technique.

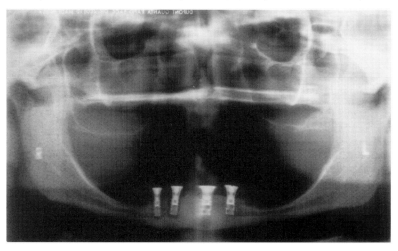

Fig. 15.8 Dental panoramic tomogram demonstrating failing implants on the right. Note the blurring of the image in the anterior region.

15.5   CONCLUSION

The choice of radiographic technique to demonstrate bone height and quantity, pre- and post implant, depends on availability of the equipment, the co-operation of the patient, and the skills of the operator.

Routine standard techniques, such as intra-oral radiographs, are applicable to dental implants as they produce images with good detail, which is necessary to assess non-existent or failing osseointegration. These are relatively easy to perform and film holders are widely available. The sophisticated tomographic techniques have advantages when a greater amount of information is required. However, the equipment is expensive and not easily accessible.

REFERENCES AND FURTHER READING

Goaz, P.W. and White, S.C. (1994). *Oral radiology — Principles and interpretation* (3rd edn) Mosby, St. Louis.

Spiekerman, H. (1995). *Color atlas of dental medicine implantology.* Georg Thieme Verlag, Stuttgard. New York Thieme Medical Publishers Inc., New York.

Frederiksen, N.L. (1995). Diagnostic imaging in dental implantology. *Oral Surg, Oral Med, Oral Radiol Endod,* **80**, 540–54.

Horner, K. *et al.* (1996). Potential medico-legal implications of computed radiography. *British Dental Journal,* **180, No 7**, 271–3.

Albrktsson, R., Zarb, P., Worthington, P., Ericsson, R.A. (186). The long-term efficacy of currently used dental implants: A review and proposed criteria of success. *International Journal of Oral and Maxillo-Facial Implants,* **1**, 11.

16 Image quality assurance

The Ionising Radiation Regulations (IRR) of 1985 require that general dental practitioners should monitor their X-ray equipment and processing procedures at regular intervals. The concept of quality control has been recognized and undertaken in hospital X-ray departments for some considerable time. It is understood to be an essential management responsibility to maintain a high standard of radiography and to avoid wastage of film and chemicals. Such quality control allows the staff to be employed effectively, to ensure diagnostic results with minimum dose, and, overall, to budget as economically as possible.

All these factors are equally important in general dental practice, but on a smaller scale. The objectives are to produce diagnostic radiographs with the minimum of radiation to the patient, and to be cost effective. Measures for quality assurance employed in a dental practice should include:

(1) staff training;
(2) an audit of radiographs, to determine errors and reasons for errors, so these can be corrected;
(3) monitoring processing facilities for regular cleaning and changing of chemicals;
(4) monitoring the X-ray equipment and films.

The following areas for analysis should be considered:

- X-ray apparatus
- film image quality
- processing quality
- the patient
- radiographic techniques
- practice management.

16.1   X-RAY APPARATUS

First, it is worth considering how old the apparatus is and whether, as well as giving reliable results, it meets the current legislation requirements. Older apparatus do not always have such efficient mains compensators, so they are more susceptible to fluctuations in the mains supply. Older timers, in particular the clockwork ones, are not accurate enough for the short exposure time needed for the present-day fast films.

Secondly, the apparatus should produce good quality radiographs with, for example, adequate detail as well as contrast. Apparatus operating at very low kilovoltages do not demonstrate a wide range of density differentials, and also give large radiation skin doses. High kilovoltages — over 60 kVp — will need a longer anode–film distance, and give the choice of different periapical techniques without enlargement.

With the new regulations (IRR 1985 and 1988), all apparatus must be monitored regularly, and at least once every three years. Regular servicing will uncover faults at an earlier stage, for example, timer accuracy. With dental panoramic tomography apparatus, regular servicing is essential to maintain the efficiency and accuracy of the engineering. Frequency of servicing depends upon the workload, but certainly should be carried out once a year.

16.2   FILM IMAGE QUALITY

1. Intra-oral films
Different speed films — for example, for bitewings, a fast film one side and a standard speed film on the other side — should be tested and assessed for information required, diagnosis value, and lack of definition. At higher kilovoltages, faster film, with a smaller overall exposure, can be perceived to have more contrast.

2. Storage
Proper storage and stock control should be in operation for all radiographic films used. They should be kept in a cool, dry place away from ionizing radiation and chemicals.

3. Film intensifying screen combinations
If it is at all possible, try to have different combinations demonstrated. Most film companies, for example, Kodak, will give advice on any aspect of dose reduction, film screen combination, and processing. There are films with a greater latitude, to use with faster screens. This increases the margin of error for exposure exactitude.

4. Cassettes
Cassettes should be cleaned regularly with an anti-static cleaning solution. They need to be checked for light leakage — place a loaded cassette in a well-lit area for a few minutes, then process the film. If

Key points

Objectives of quality assurance
1. To reduce the radiation dose to the patients and staff
2. To reduce repeat radiographs
3. To avoid wastage
4. To reduce costs
5. To improve quality of radiographs

X-ray apparatus
1. Regular servicing of equipment by qualified engineers to check timer accuracy, tube voltage, and so on
2. Regular electrical safety checks

Film image quality
1. Use fastest film consistent with good quality
2. Store all film in a cool, dark place away from chemicals and radiation
3. Ensure proper stock control is in operation
4. Handle all films carefully
5. Cassettes should be tested for light leakage and film/screen contact, and be cleaned regularly

there are any leaks in the cassette, the film will have some fogging on it (see Fig. 16.6).

5. Film contact

The contact of the film and the screens also needs to be checked. This is done by placing an unexposed film and a sheet of graph paper in a cassette, exposing the film with a short exposure time, and then processing. If there is poor film/screen contact, this shows up as a lack of definition on the image.

6. Background fog

All films have a characteristic background fog, but this will increase with age and conditions of storage. Proper storage and stock control should be in operation for all radiographic films used – they should be kept in a cool, dry place away from ionizing radiation and chemicals (see Fig. 16.5).

7. Exposure factors

It is only possible to adjust the exposure factors if the kilovoltage is variable.

16.3   PROCESSING QUALITY (SEE CHAPTER 3)

This is an area in general dental practice which has often been criticized — the average standard of processing is low. This may be because the dentist does not become sufficiently involved, and bad practice is handed down from one employee to another. Fortunately, processing lends itself easily to problem solving.

1. For accurate quality control, a small step wedge should be employed. They may be bought commercially or made from 2 mm aluminium strips, joined to make six or seven steps (see Fig. 16.1).

2. Where the work-load is large — in the region of 300 intra-oral and 50 panoramic films per week — then the chemicals should be changed every week, or two, and the water should be changed daily.

3. An adequate number of periapical films, straight from a new packet, can be exposed at one time with the same exposure conditions.

4. These films should be kept in a light-tight box and processed at the same time, daily, or every other day. The initial film should be processed when the chemical baths have been freshly made, and in the middle of a working session.

5. In small practices, where the chemicals are changed less frequently, these pre-exposed films would suffer latent image fading.

6. It is recommended that when keeping the same exposure conditions, a new film should be taken, and processed, once or twice a week.

7. The films should be carefully labelled and kept in a safe place, and any change in quality noted. This will show when the developer has deteriorated and needs to be replaced.

8. When the density of the step wedge has altered by one step, it is time to change the developer in non-replenishing processing.

9. If the developer is self-replenishing, then the temperature should be checked, or the developing bath changed. This difference on the step-wedge is equivalent to a loss of processing activity of one-seventh and would affect the radiation exposure factors (see Fig. 16.2).

16.3.1   Light leakage

Regular checks should be made in the dark-room for white light leakage from doors, windows, and the safe lights. The processor should also be checked that it is not letting in light.

16.3.2   Manual processing (see Ch. 3)

The faults in this method are usually very basic:

- temperature of developer too low (see Fig. 16.3)
- chemical baths not replenished (see Fig. 16.9)
- developer exhausted
- insufficient fixing
- fixer exhausted, with too high silver content
- improper washing

16.3.3   Automatic processing (see Ch. 3)

Fault analysis is more difficult with automatic processing, particularly when the cycle is automatically adjusted for temperature and replenishment of chemicals. However, the following represents part of a list of identifiable problems and possible causes:

Problem	Possible cause
(1) Low-density image.	Thermostat inaccurate — developer temperature below normal.

> **Key points**
>
> *Processing quality*
> 1. Chemicals should be changed regularly
> 2. Where applicable, the replenishment rate must be checked
> 3. Water should be changed daily
> 4. Dark-room, checked for light leakage
> 5. Regular cleaning of the processors and equipment is essential

Replenishing not efficient — this will apply when not automatically controlled and the tank levels are too low (see Fig. 16.3).

(2) High-density image — Temperature of developer too high, (see Fig. 16.4). Developer contamination.

(3) Film fogging. — Light fogging when film introduced into the processor (see Fig. 16.12). Light too strong through window (see Fig. 16.11).

(4) Marks and scratching — Damaged or dirty rollers, (see Fig. 16.15), Water contamination.

(5) Improperly fixed film — Wrong film type, Rate of replenishment of level of fixers too low, Silver content too high, Temperature of fixer too low.

(6) Improperly dried film — Water supply not turned on, Drier faulty, Developer or fixer replenishment rate too low, Contamination of chemicals.

16.4 THE PATIENT

1. Variations in the density must be taken into account, as these demonstrate variations in the patient's anatomy.
2. If old films are available, these can give useful information.
3. Co-operation of the patient is essential (see Fig. 16.19).
4. With children, special care is needed in placing the film in the mouth and having the correct exposure factors ready for exposure as quickly as possible (see Fig. 16.18).
5. There are great differences in pain tolerance level, but discomfort and the gag reflex can cause genuine problems, so a time and motion procedure is essential (*see* p. Ch. 6).

16.5 RADIOGRAPHIC TECHNIQUE (SEE CHAPTERS 4 AND 5)

1. Consideration should be given as to which method will give most information, and whether film holders are advantageous.
2. Anatomical configurations can limit the choice of techniques.
3. The operator's competence and level of experience may affect the quality of the radiograph.

16.6 PRACTICE MANAGEMENT

Another factor in the quality control of radiographs is the general pattern of management within the practice, and how the taking and processing of radiographs fits into this, for example, whether films are processed individually, or in batches. The following are areas within management control and responsibility:

- workload
- operator, for example, dentist or auxiliary staff
- training, if necessary, in diagnostic techniques and protection rules
- film and chemical stock control
- equipment maintenance
- methods of quality control, assessment, and correction
- effective use of quality assurance to control costing.

There are many ways in which the quality of radiographs in general dental practice could be monitored and improved. In view of the Ionising Radiation Regulations (1985 and 1988), the dentist should consider seriously how to do this. Here is a suggested quality control routine to undertake over a one-week span:

(1) Monitor details of all patients radiographed:
    (a) technique and area employed
    (b) number of films taken
    (c) exact exposure factors (including distance)
    (d) anatomical problem, if any
    (e) patient's age
    (f) operator's name
(2) Processing:
    (a) start with new chemical baths
    (b) monitor conditions every day — temperature, level of tanks
    (c) process control films daily, at the same time

Key points

- Old films should be available
- Variations in the patients anatomy must be taken into account
- Co-operation and consent of the patient is essential
- Time and motion procedure essential
- Operator competence may effect quality of radiograph
- General pattern of pratice management may effect quality control
- Monitor details of each patient radiographed
- Assess processing
- Perform reject film analysis

(3) Reject film analysis:

Keep all films, even rejections, and analyse results under headings:

(a) processing: any fault exposure: under, correct, over radiographic: position of film (see Fig. 16.24). technique: bending of film (see Fig. 16.26), vertical angulation (see Chapters 4 and 5, and Fig. 16.27), horizontal or lateral angulation (see Chapter 5 and Fig. 16.28), centring of beam (see Fig. 16.29).

Apart from controlling processing conditions, it is in this last area that quality assurance can be of the greatest help. This should be the responsibility of the radiation protection supervisor and could be invaluable in multiple practices.

16.7   POSTAL MONITORING SERVICE

See Chapter 1.

16.8   FILM FAULTS

Density of exposure (Figs 16.1–16.4)

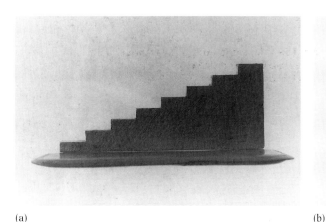 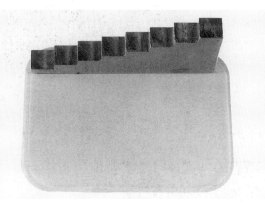

(a)   (b)

Fig. 16.1   Small step wedge on periapical film.

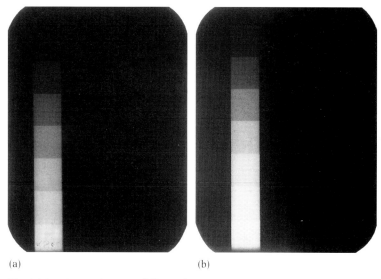

(a)   (b)

Fig. 16.2 Step wedge control films taken in a general practice: (a) with new chemicals; (b) after one week's use. Notice the deterioration in activity — the lessening of blackening down one step in the step wedge.

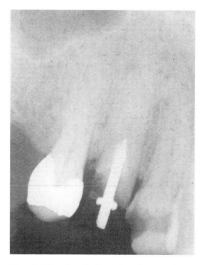

Fig. 16.3 Insufficient density may be due to underexposure; curtailed development time, the low temperature of the developer, incorrect dilution of the developer, or bleaching of the film by over fixation.

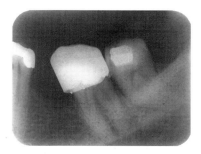

Fig. 16.4 Excessive density may be due to overexposure; excessive development time; or the high temperature of the developer.

Pre-processing faults *(Figs 16.5–16.8)*

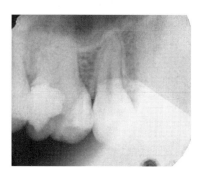

Fig. 16.5 Fogging may be due to leakage of white light in the dark-room or processing unit; faulty safe lighting; excessively long development time; bad storage conditions (damp or hot); use of film after expiry date; or films not protected from X-rays before exposure (as above).

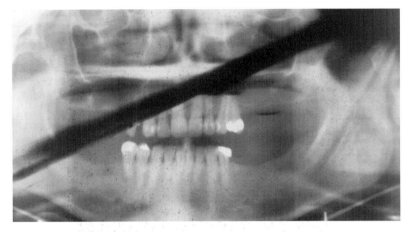

Fig. 16.6   Light leakage into cassette, fogging the film.

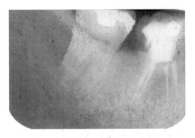

Fig. 16.7   Imprint of the finger due to insufficient drying of the hands before unwrapping of the film.

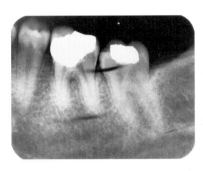

Fig. 16.8   Finger-nail marks made by the patient holding the film; the operator bending film; or the dark-room technician bending the film while opening the film packet.

Manual processing faults *(Figs 16.9 and 16.10)*

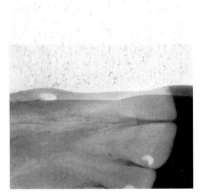

Fig. 16.9   Blank portion of the film caused by the low level of the developing solution in the tank.

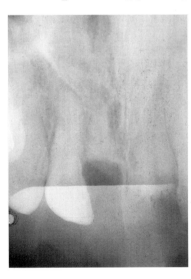

Fig. 16.10   Lack of detail in area of film where films have been in contact during development. Films must be carefully clipped on to the hanger without overlapping.

Automatic processing faults (Figs 16.11–16.15)

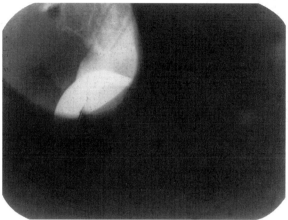

Fig. 16.11 Film fogged in daylight processor — placed in direct sunlight. Only an area protected by thumb has not been exposed to the sunlight.

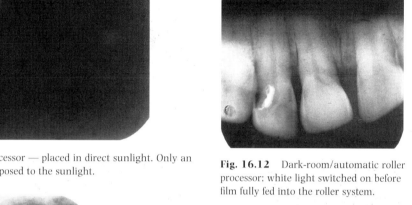

Fig. 16.12 Dark-room/automatic roller processor: white light switched on before film fully fed into the roller system.

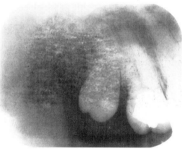

Fig. 16.13 Automatic roller processor, film fed into system with black protective paper still adjacent to film.

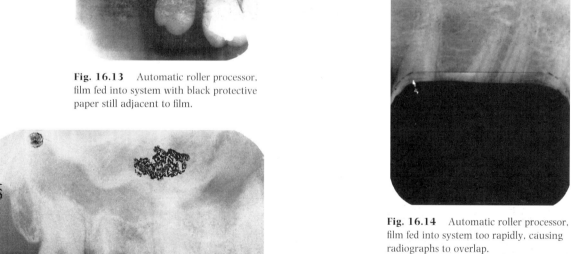

Fig. 16.14 Automatic roller processor, film fed into system too rapidly, causing radiographs to overlap.

Fig. 16.15 Automatic roller processor: marks on film from sediment caused by insufficient cleaning of rollers.

General processing faults (Fig. 16.16)

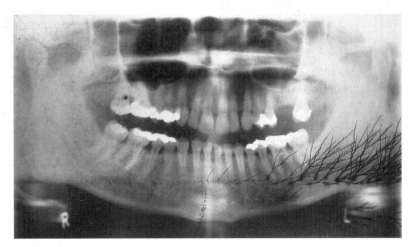

Fig. 16.16   Static mark caused by removal of the film too rapidly from the cassette.

Patient (Figs 16.17–16.21)

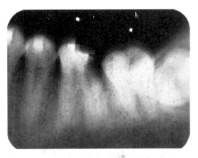

Fig. 16.17   Blurring of the image may be due to the movement of the patient and film; or the movement of the X-ray tube.

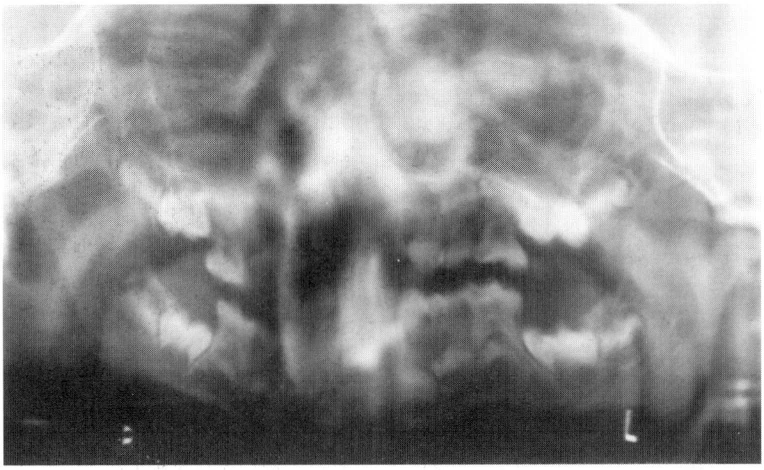

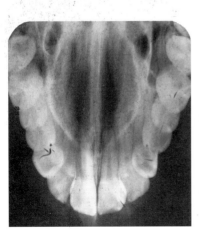

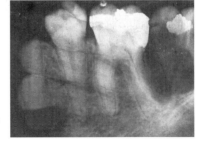

Fig. 16.18   Dental panoramic tomogram demonstrating movement during the exposure.

Fig. 16.19   Pressure marks due to patient biting too hard on to film.

Fig. 16.20   Double exposure due to carelessness of the operator.

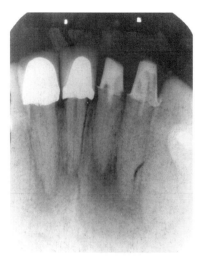

Fig. 16.21 Film demonstrating (a) pressure marks due to nail; (b) line below right central incisor, which might have represented a fracture, made by trying to bend the film into the arch.

Technique faults (Figs 16.22–16.28)

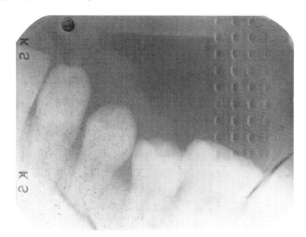

Fig. 16.22 Film placed in the mouth back to front. The foil absorbed some radiation and the characteristic imprint is demonstrated. The black lines in the lower corners demonstrate the pressure marks due to bending the film.

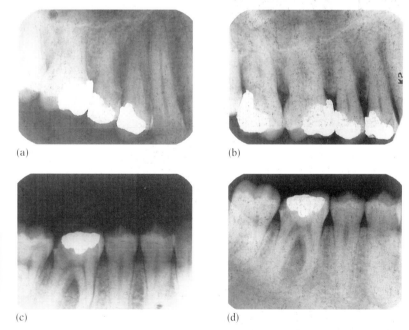

(a)

(b)

(c)

(d)

Fig. 16.24 Position of film: (a) lower border of film not level with crowns in upper molars — apex not demonstrated; (b) correctly placed — note the expanded area of rarefaction associated with palatal root of first molar; (c) film not placed deep enough into the floor of the mouth — apex not demonstrated; (d) correctly placed — demonstrating periodontal infection at the bifurcation extending to the apex.

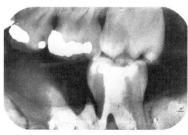

Fig. 16.23 Damage to the film due to excessive saliva seeping into the film packet, when the film was not dried after removal from the mouth.

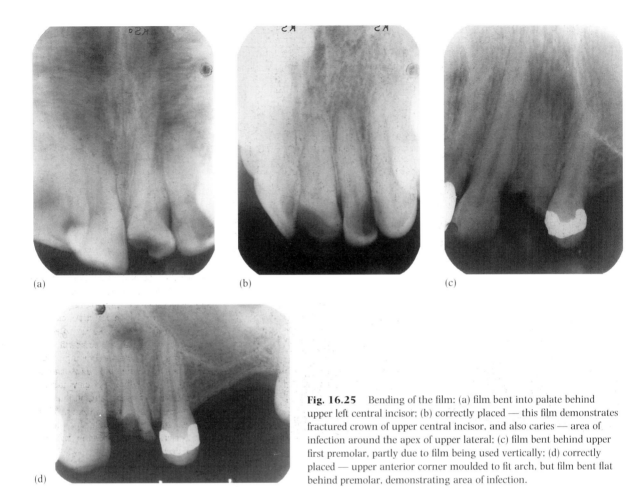

(a)

(b)

(c)

(d)

Fig. 16.25 Bending of the film: (a) film bent into palate behind upper left central incisor; (b) correctly placed — this film demonstrates fractured crown of upper central incisor, and also caries — area of infection around the apex of upper lateral; (c) film bent behind upper first premolar, partly due to film being used vertically; (d) correctly placed — upper anterior corner moulded to fit arch, but film bent flat behind premolar, demonstrating area of infection.

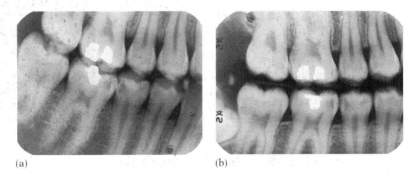

(a)

(b)

Fig. 16.26 (a) Bitewing radiograph with an upper angulation of the X-ray beam to the occlusal plane. (b) Bitewing with correct angulation. Though it is possible to diagnose caries in the lower teeth with (a), the interstitial caries between 5/ and 6/ could easily be missed.

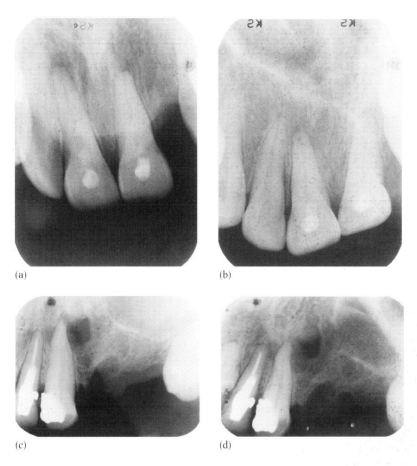

(a)   (b)

(c)   (d)

Fig. 16.27 Lateral angulation: (a) apex of upper right central not clearly demonstrated — overlapping lateral; (b) correct X-ray beam direction, clearly demonstrating area of infection solely around upper lateral; (c) periapical radiography of /3 region showing area of translucency which could be associated with the canine; (d) further view taken with a change of lateral angulation, centring over the premolar region. This separates the area of translucency which was, in fact, the result of the extraction of an apicectomied /4.

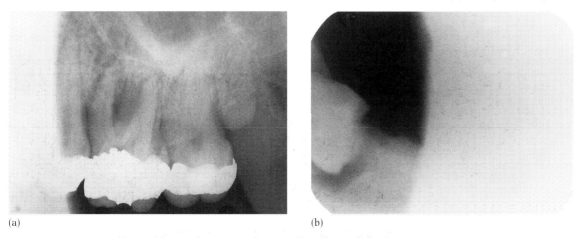

(a)   (b)

Fig. 16.28 Centring of beam: (a) X-ray beam correctly centred but film not behind horizontal third molar; (b) film correctly positioned but X-ray beam not covering film because it is centred too posteriorly.

REFERENCES AND FURTHER READING

Manson Hing, L.R. (1985). *Fundamentals of dental radiography* (2nd edn.) Lea and Febiger, St Louis.

Jenkins, D. (1980). *Radiographic photography and imaging processes.* MTP Press Ltd, Lancaster.

Hewitt, J.M. (1984). *The development and operation of a method for the remote determination of X-ray parameters used in dental radiography R 164.* National Radiation Protection Board (NRPB).

Thorogood, J., Horner, K., and Smith, N.J.D. (1988). Quality control in processing of dental radiographs — a practical guide to sensitometry. *British Journal of Radiography.*

Horner, K. (1992). Quality assurance: 1 Reject analysis, operator technique, and the X-Ray set. *Dental Update*, **19**, 75–80.

Horner, K. (1992). Quality assurance: 2 The image receptor, the darkroom, and processing. *Dental Update*, **19**, 120–6.

Starritt, H.C. *et al.* (1994). *Quality assurance in dental radiology. The Institute of Physical Sciences in Medicine, report no. 67.*

Index